New Advances in Neglected Tropical Diseases

Edited by Márcia Aparecida Sperança

Published in London, United Kingdom

New Advances in Neglected Tropical Diseases
http://dx.doi.org/10.5772/intechopen.98019
Edited by Márcia Aparecida Sperança

Contributors
Ricardo Dantas Luiz Dantas Machado, Luciane Moreno Storti-Melo, Andrea Regina de Souza Baptista, Gustavo Capatti Cassiano, Michael S. Avumegah, Isabela Ramos, Fabio Gomes, Alfonso J. Rodriguez-Morales, D. Katterine Bonilla-Aldana, María de la Soledad Lagunes Castro, Aracely López-Monteon, Daniel Guzmán-Gómez, Angel Ramos-Ligonio, Márcia Aparecida Sperança, Max Mario Fuhlendorf, Carla Moreira Santana, Felipe Baena Garcia, Aline Diniz Cabral, Ângela Maria Lorenço, Cristiane Castro Faccini, Abílio Augusto Fragata Filho, Edmar Silva Santos

First published in London, United Kingdom, 2023 by IntechOpen
IntechOpen is the global imprint of INTECHOPEN LIMITED, registered in England and Wales, registration number: 11086078, 5 Princes Gate Court, London, SW7 2QJ, United Kingdom

British Library Cataloguing-in-Publication Data
A catalogue record for this book is available from the British Library

Additional hard and PDF copies can be obtained from orders@intechopen.com

New Advances in Neglected Tropical Diseases
Edited by Márcia Aparecida Sperança
p. cm.
Print ISBN 978-1-80355-345-0
Online ISBN 978-1-80355-346-7
eBook (PDF) ISBN 978-1-80355-347-4

Meet the editor

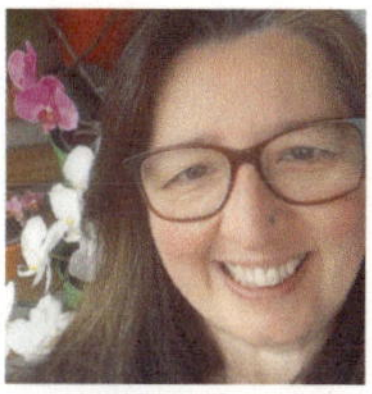

Márcia Aparecida Sperança is an Associate Professor at the Center for Natural and Human Sciences of Universidade Federal do ABC (UFABC, São Bernardo do Campo, São Paulo, Brazil). After obtaining a Ph.D. in the biology of parasite-host interaction from the Parasitology Department of the Biomedical Institute of University of São Paulo, Dr. Sperança worked as an assistant professor and researcher at Marilia Medical School, São Paulo. Her scientific expertise is in diagnosis, molecular biology, and epidemiology of arboviruses, the bacteria *Helicobacter pylori*, malaria parasites, Chagas disease, leishmaniasis and COVID-19. Since 2009, Dr. Sperança has headed the Laboratory of Pathogenic Agents at UFABC, whose multi- and interdisciplinary academic interests are characteristics of her fields of investigation.

Contents

Preface

According to the World Health Organization (WHO), neglected tropical diseases (NTDs) comprise 20 conditions, whose etiological agents include arboviruses such as dengue and Chikungunya fever, parasitic diseases such as Chagas disease, leishmaniasis, lymphatic filariasis, and bacterial diseases such as Buruli ulcer. NTDs are associated with poverty, causing economic and social consequences by affecting population health, principally in tropical and subtropical impoverished regions of the world. Many NTDs are also associated with environmental degradation, and the infectious agents present complex life cycles, including invertebrate vectors and animal reservoirs, making their control challenging for public health institutions.

This book covers various important aspects of the fight against these complex NTDs: scientific advances in the form of new biotechnological tools to promote their diagnosis, control and treatment; knowledge of their eco-epidemiology and physiopathology to promote efficient interventions to block transmission and treat diseases; and characterization of molecular targets to be employed in the development of diverse control and treatment strategies.

In the first section of the book, the first chapter reviews the literature on the use of digital PCR (ddPCR) and next-generation sequencing (NGS) to diagnose NTDs and to identify hosts and reservoirs of a variety of pathogens, thus helping in the characterization of their complex life cycles. A second chapter, which includes new findings on insects' reproductive biology, considers how this information can be used in vector control strategies. The eco-epidemiology of arboviruses in Latin America and the physiopathology of Burili ulcer disease caused by *Mycobacterium ulcerans* are the subjects of the second section. The third section contains two chapters that describe two molecular targets, the circumsporozoite protein (CSP) from the malaria parasite *Plasmodium vivax,* and an ecotin-like serine protease inhibitor of *Trypanosoma cruzi* (TcISP2), the agent of Chagas disease.

This book contributes to knowledge on new advances in NTDs and will inspire a broad public to investigate these complex diseases which, according to the WHO, affect more than one billion people globally. I am grateful to all the authors for their important contributions and to IntechOpen for once more allowing me the privilege of editing a book of high scientific value that will make a decisive contribution to tackling serious global public health problems.

Márcia Aparecida Sperança
Centro de Ciâncias Naturais e Humanas,
Universidade Federal do ABC,
São Bernardo do Campo, São Paulo, Brazil

Section 1

Diagnosis and Vector Control

Chapter 1

Metabarcoding and Digital PCR (dPCR): Application in the Study of Neglected Tropical Diseases

María de la Soldedad Lagunes-Castro, Aracely López-Monteon, Daniel Guzmán-Gómez and Angel Ramos-Ligonio

Abstract

Neglected tropical diseases such as Chagas disease, dengue, Zika, chikungunya, and malaria cause millions of deaths each year and they are caused by a variety of pathogens whose diagnosis is very limited or subject to conventional testing, making a treatment less accessible, accurate and timely diagnosis for choosing their treatments. Traditional methods for pathogen detection have not been able to meet the growing need for diagnosis and control. The incorporation of new technologies such as next-generation sequencing (NGS) and digital PCR (dPCR) represent a better diagnostic possibility due to their ability to absolutely quantify pathogens with high selectivity and precision. Our planet is currently experiencing environmental changes of an unprecedented magnitude and rate, including climate change, globalized pollution, biodiversity loss, and land use changes, so neglected diseases require a comprehensive understanding of the ecology of vectors in the different eco-epidemiological contexts, as well as of the transmission cycles of pathogens and their transmission dynamics. In this sense, NGS and dPCR open a new panorama for a better understanding of these diseases with the aim of proposing new programs for their care.

Keywords: neglected tropical diseases (NTDs), DNA, metabarcoding, dPCR, next-generation sequencing (NGS), diagnosis, pathogen detection, digital droplet PCR (ddPCR), ecohealth

1. Introduction

Neglected tropical diseases (NTDs) can be caused by viruses, bacteria, parasites, fungi, and toxins. They occur mainly in tropical areas of 149 countries on the planet, mainly concentrated in Africa and Latin America, and are called "neglected" because at the political, health, and research levels, what is necessary has not been done to eliminate them, and, furthermore, the money allocated to serving them is practically nil. According to the World Health Organization (WHO), there are 20 NTDs and one-sixth of the world's population suffers from at least one of these diseases [1, 2]. The majority of the affected population live in poor socioeconomic conditions, with low income, low educational level, and precarious housing where, in addition to the beliefs, attitudes and behaviors of these people cause social exclusion. NTDs predominate in tropical and humid climates, mainly in rural areas, conflict zones, and regions of difficult access. However, urban areas can also be affected. The presence of these diseases has been increasing due to factors such as climate change [3–5]. The absence of timely and accurate diagnoses, quality medical care, medicines, vaccines, and access to drinking water and sanitation services are the factors that increase the presence of NTDs and can only be faced with leadership and political effort economic as a whole since they do not top the list of priorities in public health policies. The development in the research of new and better medicines and diagnostic methods by the industry is very scarce. In addition, reliable statistical data makes it difficult for these diseases to be known by society [6–9].

These diseases are of increasing concern, as the geographic range of tropical diseases is expanding due to climate change, urbanization, changing agricultural practices, deforestation, and biodiversity loss [10]. Infectious diseases can be unpredictable with the potential risk of global outbreaks. However, the way we characterize pathogens has changed dramatically. Although increasingly sophisticated diagnostic tools have improved the ability to detect the presence of the pathogens that cause these diseases, this ability comprises only a small part of the set of tools necessary to generate an accurate etiological diagnosis to manage these health threats. For this, the ecoepidemiology of diseases must be taken into account, with an approach to the interdependence of individuals and their connection with the levels of individual, social, molecular, and environmental organization that participate in the causal processes of diseases [11, 12]. Over the years, molecular methods have evolved and improved, from conventional endpoint polymerase chain reaction (PCR) to real-time quantitative PCR (qPCR), DNA microarrays, digital droplet PCR (ddPCR), loop-mediated isothermal amplification (LAMP), and metagenomic approaches based on high-throughput next-generation DNA sequencing (HT-NGS). Such technological achievements have contributed to expanding the set of analytical tools used to solve various research objectives, including disease diagnosis. The next-generation sequencing (NGS) has generated a trigger in the discovery and characterization of pathogens, leaving behind old culture methods and techniques and making it possible to detect non-culturable pathogens that were previously difficult to diagnose. On the other hand, due to its sensitivity and quantitative characteristics, digital polymerase chain reaction (dPCR) is a potential candidate to become an attractive new method among molecular technologies for parasite detection and quantitative analysis, favoring a better understanding of the transmission dynamics of the pathogens that cause these diseases [13–18].

2. Next generation sequencing (NGS)

2.1 DNA sequencing: history and current status

The description of the molecular structure of DNA in 1953 by Watson and Crick, reported in their article "molecular structure of nucleic acids: A structure for deoxyribose nucleic acid" [19], became the basis of genomic research allowing technological development and research. At the beginning of the 70s, studies on DNA sequencing began, Maxam and Gilbert in February 1977 stated that DNA can be sequenced by a chemical procedure [20]. However, the first enzymatic method for DNA sequencing was proposed by Sanger and Coulson in 1975 [21]. In 1982, Caruthers and Hood developed the first automated method for sequencing DNA [22], which was capable of sequencing fragments from 5 to 75 base pairs (bp), and in 1986, Hood and Smith designed the first automatic sequencer that used laser beams that recognize fluorescent markers on DNA [23–25]. By 1985, the first automated sequencers using gels (Applied Biosystems PRISM® 373) or polymer-coated capillaries (ABI PRISM® 310) appeared [26]. Later, in 2004, new sequencing methods emerged, based on pyrosequencing and the so-called next generation sequencing (NGS) platforms. Currently, due to the fact that new sequencers have appeared on the market that are capable of applying other sequencing technologies in parallel, it is more appropriate to speak of High-Throughput Sequencing (HTS) or massive sequencing. There are some variants of this technology such as sequencing by ligation (*sequencing by oligonucleotide ligation and detection*), sequencing by synthesis and semiconduction, and sequencing by synthesis in clusters (sequence length up to 600 bp). A third generation of sequencers is those that use single molecule sequencing (*single molecule real-time* [SMRT]) that allows sequencing of much longer molecules, up to 30 kb [27–29]. There are other sequencing technologies in the development phase, those based on nanopores; which are based on the identification of the different bases of the DNA chain, thanks to an optical signal or by the variation that occurs in an electric current when the chain passes through a nanopore anchored to a membrane, in situ nucleic acid sequencing; which is a progression of single-cell RNA sequencing methods, is performed intracellularly within intact tissues, thus preserving the spatial context of gene expression within and between cell types and sequencing based on direct observation with microscopy that uses electron microscopy and allows the DNA sequence to be read directly by optical methods without the need for amplification (**Figure 1**) [30, 31] .

2.2 Inside to the NSG methodology

High-throughput DNA sequencing techniques are capable of sequencing a large number of different DNA sequences in a single reaction, which is why they are also

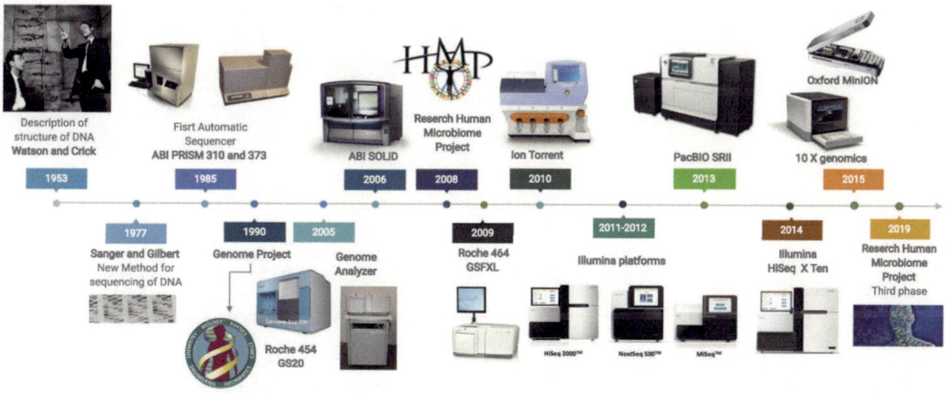

Figure 1.
Sequencing technology timeline. Research in DNA sequencing technologies is in continuous development. In the last decade, NGS tests have established their value as a diagnostic test, given their good performance for the detection of genetic diseases and the discovery of new pathogenic variants. This technology has facilitated molecular diagnosis, being a more efficient and faster tool in gene sequencing, and has facilitated the identification and classification of multiple genetic variants together with their respective pathological association. Additionally, the costs of sequencing and the duration in which the diagnosis is defined have been reduced, which allows timely prevention measures to be established in patients with high risk in the future.

known as "next generation" and "massive parallel" DNA sequencing. In general, the material to be sequenced is double-stranded DNA; however, genomic DNA, reverse transcribed RNA or cDNA, immunoprecipitated DNA can be used [32]. Nucleic acid templates are first prepared for sequencing (library generation), this step differs according to the platform to be used. For a short read, three steps generally apply: (1) fragmentation of DNA to application-specific template lengths, (2) ligation of adapters to facilitate attachment of fragments to solid surfaces (such as microchips, microspheres, or nanowells) or to circularize, and (3) amplification of templates for provide enough copies of each template to allow the sequencer to detect them. Libraries can be read from one end only (single-ended read), or from both ends (double-ended reads). Some technical errors can occur when preparing libraries that are related to the amplification and sequencing of the PCR products, mainly inherent polymerase errors and inefficiencies associated with the guanine-cytosine (GC) content of the template. To solve this, libraries have been prepared without the use of the PCR reaction for short-read platforms, increasing the fidelity of the sequence. Long read platforms do not require an amplification step.

After library preparation, which attaches adapters to approximately 450 bp DNA fragments, the templates are annealed to a glass slide bearing complementary adapters. Once attached to the solid surface, the fragments are amplified by PCR from either one end or both ends, producing billions of sets of DNA fragments from the clonal template that can be sequenced simultaneously. Raw obtained sequence reads are typically set to FASTQ format [33]. Subsequently, the sequences are aligned with a reference genome using an alignment tool [34] in order to obtain a map file of the sequence alignment (read assembly and base sequence) (**Figure 2**). A typical whole genome sequence will produce on the order of 5 million SNVs and 250,000 short

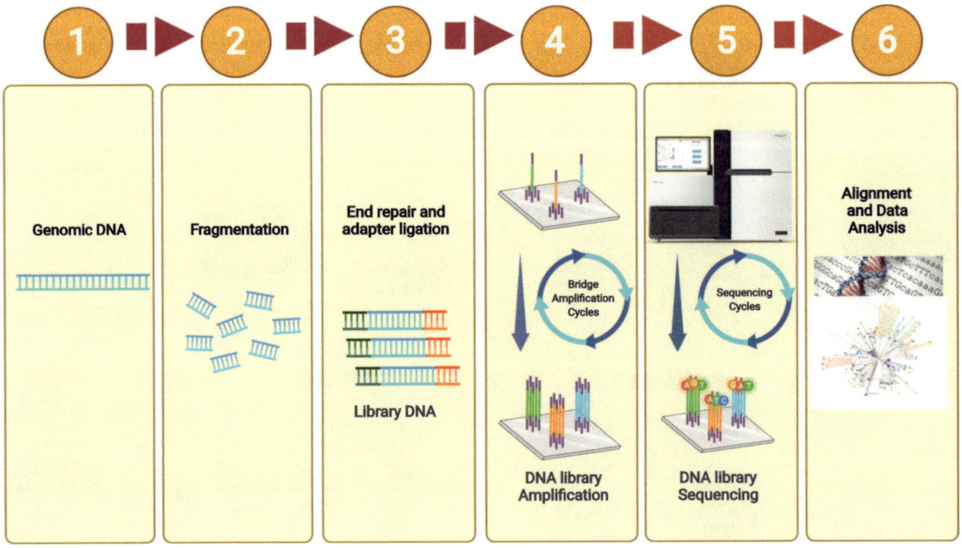

Figure 2.
Next generation sequencing (NGS) is a group of technologies designed to sequence large numbers of DNA segments massively and in parallel, in less time and at a lower cost per base. The methodological approach can be summarized in five steps: 1) segmentation of the DNA into several fragments, 2) labeling of the DNA by means of primers or adapters that indicate the starting point for replication, 3) amplification of the DNA fragments labeled with adapters by methods based on polymerase chain reaction, 4) sequencing or reading of the DNA fragments, and 5) reconstruction of the complete sequence by means of reference sequences and export to data storage files.

indels. Ignoring common single nucleotide polymorphisms and short insertions or deletions (indels), there are typically about 300,000 unique variants left to consider (**Figure 2**) [31, 35, 36].

3. Digital polymerase chain reaction (dPCR)

3.1 The evolution of PCR

Since the development of the polymerase chain technique (PCR) in 1971 when Gobind Khorana described the technique by explaining the replication of a DNA fragment using two primers [37]. But it was in 1983 that Kary Mullis and his colleagues at the Californian company Cetus Corporation first carried it out while working on making oligonucleotides and using primers for DNA sequencing. Used two primers that aligned with each of the DNA strands, added *Escherichia coli* DNA polymerase I and triphosphated nucleotides. As a result, they obtained the exponential replication of the DNA fragment flanked by the primers [38]. This endpoint PCR technique has evolved thanks to two factors, the discovery of the Taq polymerase and the thermal cycler (**Figure 3**). Thus, today we can find variants such as: reverse transcription PCR (RT-PCR) [39, 40], Circularized RT-PCR (cRT-PCR) [41], inverse PCR [42], nested PCR [43], in situ PCR [44], multiplex PCR [45], multiplex-ready PCR [46], asymmetric PCR [47], Ligation-anchored PCR [48], long fragment PCR [49], Fluorescent Quantitative PCR (Real Time PCR; qPCR) [50], Immune PCR (IPCR) [51], and digital PCR (dPCR) (**Figure 3**). dPCR was first conceptualized in the 1990s. It is based on limiting dilutions, PCR and Poisson distribution [52]. dPCR is classified into digital droplet PCR (ddPCR) and digital chip PCR (cdPCR). cdPCR presents a challenge to achieve high throughput, however, ddPCR can overcome this impediment [53]. It is worth mentioning that isothermal amplification methods called LAMP (LOOP-mediated isothermal amplification) have been developed that, unlike PCR technology, amplify the target sequence at a constant temperature of 60–65°C. based on strong strand displacement DNA polymerase and 4–6 specifically designed primers can be used that can recognize and amplify six or eight regions of a given target

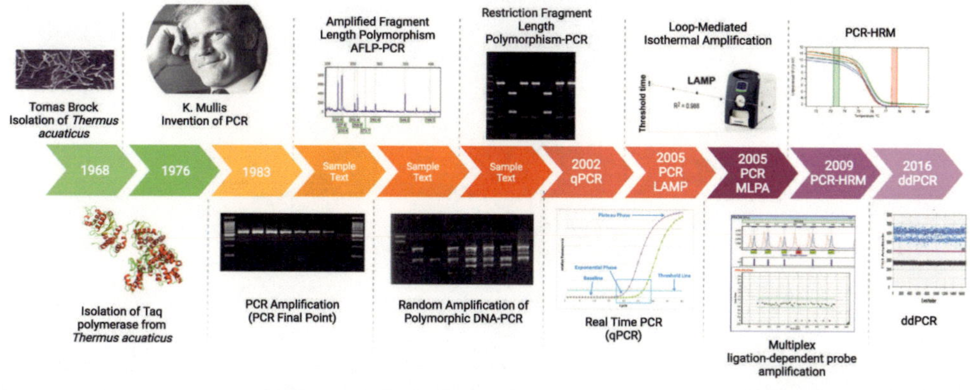

Figure 3.
Evolution of the PCR technique. PCR technology has undergone continual improvements. The applications of PCR are multiple, encompassing from the evolution to the clinic, passing through the genetics, molecular biology, and biotechnology; in addition to applications in agriculture and livestock. The applications of this new technique seem to have no limits.

gene to achieve higher analytical specificity. Amplification signals can be detected by photometry of the turbidity of the reaction or by colorimetry of the fluorescent intensity of the intercalated dyes. This approach offers a fast (1 h), a low-cost, easier-to-use, thermocycler-free alternative method for PCR [54, 55].

3.2 Principles and benefits of dPCR

The basis of ddPCR is to distribute a nucleic acid-containing sample to thousands of independent partitions. There are several ways to create these droplets: manual partitioning, immiscible liquid chemistry, atomization, etc. The generated droplets contain only one target DNA molecule or none at all [56]. To determine target DNA copies without bias, templates with target DNA must be randomly distributed and microdroplets must be produced in large numbers. These partitions can be individually amplified through thermal cycling. Unlike qPCR, which produces an exponential signal and quantifies samples by comparing their CTs (threshold cycle) to a standard curve generated by well-defined samples; by determining the concentration of the sample using an "analog" method, ddPCR technology generates linear digital signals that allow quantitative analysis of the PCR product, being able to detect very rare mutations with high precision and sensitivity, and these amplicons can be quantified without a curve standard [53]. Quantification of DNA molecules is performed by a combination of Poisson distribution and dilution templates at the single-molecule level. The number of templates correlates positively with positive wells, so the exact number of template copies can be calculated. The use of the presence and absence of signals to indicate the target DNA makes a direct "digital" measurement of the samples [57] (**Figure 4**). Furthermore, due to high pipetting handling in sample preparation and PCR conditions, even with a standard curve, the data disparity in qPCR is greater than in ddPCR. ddPCR can be used to detect low concentrations of DNA [58, 59].

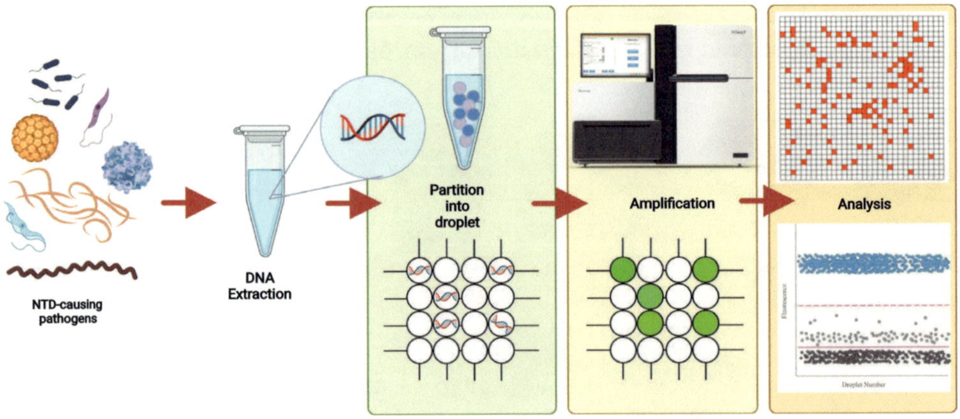

Figure 4.
Digital droplet polymerase chain reaction (ddPCR) is a highly sensitive quantitative polymerase chain reaction (PCR) method based on fractionation of the sample into thousands of individual nano-sized water-in-oil reactions. Recently, ddPCR has become one of the most accurate and sensitive instruments for DNA detection. Consists of simple steps to follow: 1) prepare PCR-ready samples before starting ddPCR, 2) droplet generation, 3) droplet amplification by PCR; 4) Reading of drops, and 5) analysis of results. Positive droplets, which contain at least one copy of the target, exhibit greater fluorescence than negative droplets.

4. Uses of NSG and dPCR in the diagnosis of the causal agents of NTDs

NTDs are caused by several types of common and rare pathogens. A common concern with conventional testing methods is the limitation in the range of pathogens that can be detected and the lack of sensitivity for their diagnosis. Obstacles such as incomplete knowledge of natural history make it difficult to understand the ecology and pathogenesis of rare and neglected diseases. Emerging technologies, including NGS and dPCR, provide opportunities to accelerate the diagnosis and development of treatments for these diseases [60, 61]. The application of NGS in Leishmania isolates has allowed the characterization of populations through the identification and analysis of variations. Information on population structure can reveal important insights into disease dynamics and identify genetic backgrounds associated with parasite virulence and ecology [62]. The metagenomic analysis of the Leishmania vectors revealed the microbiota present in them, these studies will allow us to understand how the microbiota interacts with the parasite vectors and to develop tools for biological control [63]. Also by means of NGS, it has been observed that some HLA class I and class II genes could be involved in the predisposition of cutaneous leishmaniasis [64].

Mycetoma is one of the neglected tropical diseases, characterized by painless subcutaneous inflammation, multiple paranasal sinuses, and discharge containing aggregates of the infectious organism known as pimples. Studies of host genetic variation in mycetoma susceptibility by NGS will allow the identification of new treatments for mycetoma and will also improve the ability to stratify 'at risk' individuals, allowing the possibility of developing preventive and personalized clinical care strategies in the future [65]. The application of NGS in the study of malaria has greatly contributed to a better understanding of Plasmodium biology as well as host–parasite interactions [66].

Trypanosoma cruzi, the etiological agent of Chagas disease, represents a challenge due to its repetitive nature. Only three of the parasite's six recognized discrete typing units (DTUs) have their draft genomes published, and, therefore, analyzes of genome evolution in the taxon are limited, thus the assembly of short NGS reads can be applied for the detection of highly repetitive genomes [67]. Also, single nucleotide polymorphisms (SNPs) have been identified in the protein sequences of *T. cruzi* [68] and studies have been carried out with an EcoHealth approach [69]. These results may lead to a better understanding of Chagas disease and will provide further development of biomarkers for the prognosis, diagnosis, and development of drugs for the treatment of Chagas disease.

Comparisons of *Treponema pallidum* genomic sequences using NGS have revealed a modular structure of several genomic loci. This diversification of *T. pallidum* genomes appears to be facilitated by genome recombination events within the strain [70]. On the other hand, unbiased sequencing of the Zika virus genome obtained by NGS from the cerebrospinal fluid of one patient revealed that no virus mutations associated with anatomical compartments were detected [71] and NGS has also been used in different experimental and epidemiological settings to understand how the adaptive evolution of dengue variants shapes the dengue epidemic and disease severity through its transmission [72].

ddPCR has been shown to be more accurate than qPCR; therefore, it has been finely modified to detect low-abundance nucleic acids, which might be more suitable for clinical diagnosis [59]. Human strongyloidiasis is one of the neglected tropical diseases caused by infection with soil-transmitted helminth *Strongyloides stercoralis*. Conventional stool examination, a method commonly used for diagnosis of

S. stercoralis, has low sensitivity, especially in the case of light infections. However, the use of ddPCR showed high sensitivity and specificity for the detection of *S. stercoralis* in stool samples. This technique can help improve diagnosis, especially in cases of mild infection. In addition, the ddPCR technique could be useful for the detection of patients before starting immunosuppressive drug therapy and the follow-up after treatment of strongyloidiasis [73]. The usefulness of the ddPCR platform in the detection of *T. cruzi* infection has also been evaluated. The clinical sensitivity and specificity of the assay were both 100%, with perfect agreement between positive and negative qPCR and ddPCR results in the clinical samples tested. However, the fact of not performing a calibration curve in ddPCR offers an advantage for its use in the diagnosis of *T. cruzi* [74]. Moreover, RT-ddPCR in dengue diagnosis could help harmonize DENV quantification results and improve field findings, such as identifying a DENV titer threshold that correlates with disease severity [75, 76]. The use of ddPCR to absolutely quantify human malaria parasites successfully detects *Plasmodium falciparum* and *Plasmodium vivax*, and the sensitivity of ddPCR to detect *P. falciparum* is significantly higher than qPCR [77].

NGS and ddPCR have recently shown great potential for pathogen detection, however, in a comparative study between these techniques, the results were subject to their respective limitations and strengths, the ddPCR method being more useful for rapid detection of common isolated pathogens, while the mNGS test is more appropriate for diagnosis where classical diagnostic methods (microbiological or molecular) fail to identify the causative pathogens [78]. NGS is a new technology that holds the promise of improving our ability to diagnose, interrogate, and track infectious diseases. For its part, the third generation of the PCR; ddPCR can be used to directly quantify and clonally amplify DNA, the latter has been widely used in the detection

NTD: Pathogen	Study objective*	Method	Reference
Anquilostomiasis *Necator americanus Ancylostoma duodenale*	—	—	—
Ascariosis *Ascaris lumbricoides*	Identification of repeated sequences for diagnostic use	NGS	[79]
Schistosomiasis *Schistosoma duodenale*	—	—	—
Cysticercosis *Taenia solium*	Diagnosis in cerebrospinal fluid	NGS	[80, 81]
	Identification and characterization of microsatellites		[82]
	Analysis and identification in soil samples	ddPCR	[83, 84]
Chagas disease *Trypanosoma cruzi*	Detection of *T. cruzi* infection	ddPCR	[74]
	Identification of trypanosomatid species in mammalian reservoirs, human patients, and sandfly vectors from endemic regions of leishmaniasis	NSG	[85]
	Detection of *T. cruzi*-specific antibodies		[86]
	EcoHealth/One Health approach		[69]

NTD: Pathogen	Study objective*	Method	Reference
Leishmaniasis	Identification of trypanosomatid species in mammalian reservoirs, human patients, and sandfly vectors from endemic regions of leishmaniasis	NSG	[85]
	Assembling nuclear genomes		[87]
	Antimony resistance gene analysis		[88]
	Parasite-host interaction for the search for target proteins used in prognosis and/or infection control		[89]
	Descriptive analysis of genomes		[62]
	Diagnosis from Cutaneous Leishmaniasis in patients	ddPCR	[90]
Leprosy *Mycobacterium leprae*	Detection of Infections	ddPCR	[91, 92]
	Identification of risk genes that affect susceptibility to leprosy	NSG	[93]
Trachoma *Chlamydia trachomatis*	Detecting and quantifying ocular	ddPCR	[94, 95]
Yaws *Treponema pallidum*	Subspecies identification	NSG	[96]
	Reconstruction of genomes		[97]
	Evolutionary origin		[98]
	study syphilis pathogenesis	NSG and ddPCR	[99]
Rabies Lyssavirus	Phylogenetic analysis	NSG	[100]
	Genetic and antigenetic characterization	NSG	[101]
Dracunculiasis (guinea-worm disease)	—	—	—
Buruli ulcer *Mycobacterium ulcerans*	Transcriptome analysis	NSG	[102]
	Analysis of recurrent infections due to continuous exposure		[103]
Trichuriasis *Trichuris trichiura*	Clinical diagnosis	ddPCR	[104]
Malaria *Plasmodium vivax Plasmodium falciparum*	Quantification in samples from asymptomatic patients	ddPCR	[77]
Onchocerciasis *Onchocerca volvulus*	analysis of the presence of Wolbachia	NSG	[105]
Elephantiasis (Lymphatic filariasis) *Wuchereria bancrofti, Brugia malayi*	Identification of sequences for diagnostic use	NSG	[106]
	Detection and quantification in blood samples and mosquitoes		[107]
	Differential gene expression	ddPCR	[108]
Fascioliasis *Fasciola hepatica* *Fasciola gigantica*	Identification of virulence genes	NSG	[109]
	Sequencing of the complete mitochondrial genome		[110]

NTD: Pathogen	Study objective*	Method	Reference
Sleeping sickness *Trypanosoma brucei*	Aneuploidy analysis	NSG	[111]
Dengue DENV	Quantification in clinical samples	RT-ddPCR	[75]
	Identification of viral pathogens in clinical samples from travelers	NSG	[112]
Zika ZIKZV	Detection and quantification in swimming pool water	RT-ddPCR	[113]
Chikungunya CHIKV	Identification and confirmation of pathogens in samples of known etiology	NSG	[114]
CHIKV, DENV, *P. vivax*, ZIKV	Epidemiological surveillance	NSG	[115]

**Only the papers deposited in the PubMed database are presented.*
DENV, Dengue virus, CHIKV, Chikungunya virus; ZIKV, Zika virus.

Table 1.
Use of NSG and ddPCR in the study of NTDs.

of low abundance nucleic acids, being useful in the diagnosis of infectious diseases and may be a better option than qPCR for clinical applications in the future. However, it is clear that to date there are few studies on the application of these technologies to the study of NTDs (**Table 1**).

5. NGS and dPCR as tools for understanding NTDs

Understanding health from different areas, based on the circumstances in which people are born and develop their lives, health systems, public policy, and environmental factors, among others, is to understand it from the approach proposed by Ecohealth. This comprehensive vision takes into account the diversity of factors that affect the presence or absence of any disease in humans and not only considers that people's health depends on the effects of pathogenic microorganisms or toxic substances. Ecohealth addresses what are known as social determinants of health [116, 117]. To analyze these determinants, it must be understood that there are singular, particular, and general dimensions that condition the health status of individuals and societies.

The control of NTDs requires novel visions and approaches that effectively address the determinants of transmission of a group of very diverse and complex pathologies that only share in some cases being transmitted by vector insects, but that have very different clinical characteristics. Their diagnoses require techniques of varying complexity and cost, they are transmitted in very specific contexts (urban, rural, and jungle), they affect the general population to varying degrees, their treatment varies in efficacy and cost, and control faces different technical challenges and operations that make the success of the programs very uncertain. On the other hand, frequent changes in environmental and ecological conditions, the dynamics of social and economic forces and the influence of cultural and gender determinants dominate the patterns of presentation and control of vector-borne diseases (endemic, epidemic, emergency, deletion, etc.). That is why the traditional approaches focused exclusively on the vector, based on the intensive and massive use of insecticides, with vertical programs isolated from health services and operational personnel far away or oblivious to the needs of the communities, are not having an impact on the profile epidemiology of each of the NTDs such as dengue, Chagas disease, and malaria to mention some NTDs [118, 119]. Based on these needs, the Ecohealth model emerges, incorporating a transdisciplinary approach in the study and care of DNTs, emphasizing social participation as a central actor in the solutions to these health problems, and proposes an approach to inequality of gender as an element to insert in prevention and control programs. The model demands a multi- and intersectoral vision to contain them in a sustainable manner and provides evidence to strengthen operational programs [120]. In this sense, NSG and dPCR can easily be very powerful tools for the comprehensive study of DNTs from an Ecohealth point of view. For example, using next-generation sequencing metagenomic analysis, a variety of viral families in mammals and rodents were studied, and the results obtained allowed us to know the viral community in wildlife that at a given moment could become a critical point for the development of an emerging disease [121]. Other work on the presence of enteroviruses (EV) in nonhuman primates through phylogenetic analysis revealed that one virus strain was related to human clinical isolates, suggesting zoonotic behavior [122]. Studies related to Chagas disease vectors have made it possible to analyze the blood-feeding sources of multiple species of triatomines with much greater sensitivity and also to identify multiclonal infections with *T. cruzi*, which must be taken into account to develop transmission networks and characterize the risk of human infection, eventually leading to better control of disease transmission [69, 123–125]. These studies represent a powerful approach to unravel and understand transmission dynamics at microgeographic levels of Chagas disease.

On the other hand, ddPCR, which is considered a biotechnological refinement of conventional polymerase chain reaction methods that can be used to directly quantify and clonally amplify DNA, has been widely used in the detection of low-abundance nucleic acids and is useful in diagnosing infectious diseases including

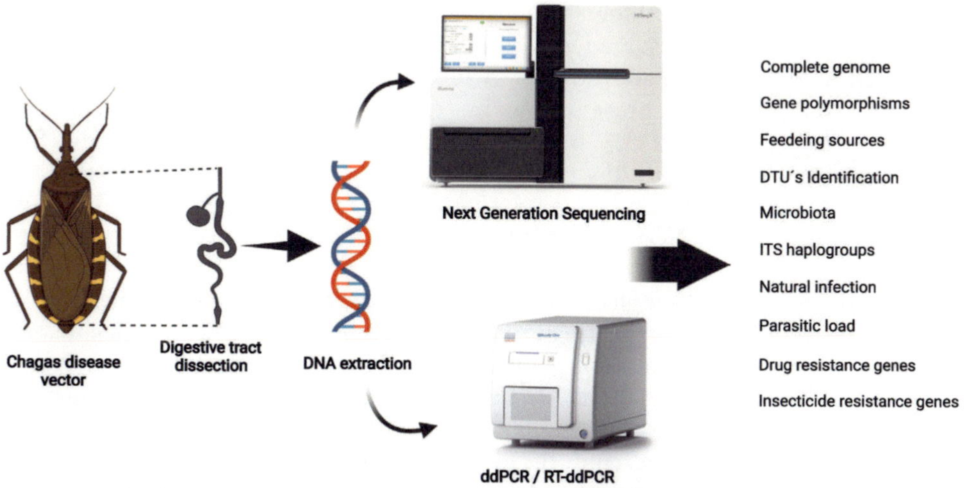

Figure 5.
The promotion of research with ecosystem approaches to human health (EcoHealth) is of great importance to contribute to improving the health of communities in the poorest regions of the world, for example, in Chagas disease, where new technologies, such as NSG and ddPCR, may have a better scope for a better understanding of the disease and thus propose new intervention policies. This strategy should be applicable to the study of all NTDs.

viral, bacterial, and parasitic infections, concluding that ddPCR provides a more sensitive, accurate, and reproducible detection of low-abundance pathogens [126, 127]. For example, Multiplex RT-ddPCR could help characterize defective genomes by simultaneously quantifying multiple regions of the same DENV RNA molecule, and in samples where quantities are limited, the application of RT-ddPCR could identify patients with burdens. Elevated viral levels, especially during the first days of the disease, could not be carried out with other methodologies due to the scarcity of the sample [75]. Therefore, the inclusion of NSG and dPCR techniques should be used jointly for the comprehensive study of NTDs so that in the future they allow the generation of interventions or sustainable strategies for vector control and transmission prevention of the NTDs (**Figure 5**).

6. Drawbacks of NSG and dPCR

One of the most common issues affecting the efficiency of NGS and dPCR is sample quality. Although platforms are often tested and compared using highly selected samples, real-life samples do not behave in the same way. Although "next generation" massively parallel DNA sequencers have been shown to offer many potential benefits in performing genetic analyses, especially for large-scale projects, one of the main drawbacks limiting their use is the relatively low error rate highly compared to standard short-read methods. In general, the main disadvantages observed in the different existing platforms are the presence of a bias in the CG ratio, high cost, and errors in the homopolymers (substitution/deletion errors in the readings) because their length is not correctly deduced from the electrical signal, the introduction of new algorithms, post-sequencing correction tools and the SNV/insertions-deletions (INDEL) tool [128], low output, short reads, and high error rate [129]. Likewise, there are also problems with long-length reads. In general, NSG and other long-read sequencing platforms suffer from a high error rate [130]. On the other hand, accuracy stands out as the most important issue for all recently developed technologies. For example, in metagenomic whole genome sequencing (mWGS), which analyzes all of the DNA or RNA in a given sample, in addition to high cost, an additional consideration for performing mWGS is the abundance of human DNA present in many types of clinical samples, such as blood and respiratory secretions [131]. Another barrier to the implementation of NGS in the diagnosis of infectious diseases has been the time it takes to complete all the steps for NGS, this turnaround time relative to conventional methods has limited the clinical relevance of NGS results for decision-making decisions about patient care [132].

On the other hand, although dPCR has numerous advantages over qPCR, it has not yet been able to fully replace the use of qPCR. It has been reported that high concentrations of nucleic acid could saturate the dPCR reaction, highlighting the importance of adequate dilution [133–136]. The low throughput compared to qPCR and the longer response times of current dPCR systems have not allowed this technique to enter routine analysis. On the other hand, the exclusivity of reagents based on the platform used is another limitation as it does not allow working with a different platform, including the multiplexing approach. Some dPCR protocols show a dynamic range similar to or smaller than that offered by a qPCR assay, which in some cases decreases the sensitivity of the assay, and lastly, the costs of equipment and reagents are still somewhat inaccessible [74, 137].

7. Conclusions

Reflecting on the public health problem that NTDs implies worldwide, improving the efficiency of the diagnosis of these pathologies is of vital importance for the development of more effective treatments. At the same time, an accurate diagnosis will limit the abusive use of drugs, thus reducing the appearance of resistance phenomena in the pathogens that cause these diseases. The traditional clinical diagnosis of infectious diseases consists of a differential analysis supported by a series of tests in order to identify the causal pathogen, which ranges from microscopic observation, the culture of microorganisms, and the detection of antibodies to the amplification of nucleic acids. Although molecular diagnostic assays are a rapid way to diagnose the most common infections, almost all current conventional microbial assays target a limited number of pathogens, these limitations mean that pathogens are not detected in up to 60% of cases and sometimes the use of cultures from clinical samples is required, where many of these pathogens are difficult to culture. Although the application of these molecular methods is a routine tool for the diagnosis of numerous diseases, they have not yet been fully used for the diagnosis of NTDs. In this sense, regardless of the current advantages and disadvantages of NGS and dPCR, these techniques have a promising application to contribute to an improvement in the diagnosis of NTDs, since they provide rapid results, allow the determination of parasitaemia in asymptomatic infections and low density, as well as the detection of pathogens difficult to cultivate. Both techniques have a higher sensitivity than conventional techniques used for diagnosis. However, more evaluations are needed, and especially the development of studies that combine NSG and dPCR technologies for the generation of comprehensive knowledge that allows a better understanding of NTDs in different ecoepidemiological contexts, as well as in the dynamics of the transmission cycles of the pathogens that cause these diseases and thus meet the goals, intermediate measures, and indicators of the roadmap on neglected tropical diseases 2021–2030 to prevent, control, and eliminate NTDs.

Acknowledgements

We thank Montserrat Ramos-López for reviewing the language. All the images you will show in this work were created with BioRender.com

Conflict of interest

The authors declare no conflict of interest.

Author details

María de la Soldedad Lagunes-Castro[1], Aracely López-Monteon[1,2], Daniel Guzmán-Gómez[1] and Angel Ramos-Ligonio[1,2]*

1 Universidad Veracruzana, Faculty of Chemical Sciences, LADISER Immunology and Molecular Biology, Orizaba, Veracruz, Mexico

2 Chagas Association with Science and Knowledge A.C. Orizaba, Veracruz, Mexico

*Address all correspondence to: angramos@uv.mx

References

[1] Pan American Health Organization (PAHO). Neglected, Tropical and Vector Borne Diseases [Internet]. 2022. Avalaible from: https://www.paho.org/en/topics/neglected-tropical-and-vector-borne-diseases

[2] Hotez PJ, Alvarado M, Basáñez M-G, et al. The global burden of disease study 2010: Interpretation and implications for the neglected tropical diseases. PLoS Neglected Tropical Diseases. 2014;**7**:e2865

[3] Conteh L, Engels T, Molyneux DH. Socioeconomic aspects of neglected tropical diseases. Lancet. 2010;**375**:239-247

[4] Joshi G, Quadir SS, Yadav KS. Road map to the treatment of neglected tropical diseases: Nanocarriers interventions. Journal of Controlled Release. 2021;**339**:51-74. DOI: 10.1016/j.jconrel.2021.09.020

[5] Booth M. Climate change and the neglected tropical diseases. Advances in Parasitology. 2018;**100**:39-126. DOI: 10.1016/bs.apar.2018.02.001

[6] King CH, Bertino AM. Asymmetries of poverty: Why global burden of disease valuations underestimate the burden of neglected tropical diseases. PLoS Neglected Tropical Diseases. 2008;**2**:e209

[7] Engels D. Neglected tropical diseases in the sustainable development goals. Lancet. 2016;**387**:223-234

[8] United Nations. A New Global Partnership: Eradicate Poverty and Transform Economies through Sustainable Development. The Reportof the High-Level Panel of Eminent Persons on the Post-2015 Development Agenda. New York: United Nations Publications; 2013

[9] Gyapong JO, Gyapong M, Yellu N, Anakwah K, Amofah G, Bockarie M, et al. Integration of control of neglected tropical diseases into health-care systems: Challenges and opportunities. Lancet. 2010;**375**(9709):160-165. DOI: 10.1016/S0140-6736(09)61249-6

[10] Zumla A, Ustianowski A. Tropical diseases: Definition, geographic distribution, transmission, and classification. Infectious Disease Clinics of North America. 2012;**2**:195-205. DOI: 10.1016/j.idc.2012.02.007.), 10.1016/j.idc.2012.02.007.)

[11] Stevenson M, Halpin K. Emerging and endemic zoonotic diseases: Surveillance and diagnostics. Revue Scientifique et Technique. 2021;**40**(1):119-129. DOI: 10.20506/rst.40.1.3212

[12] Bizouarn P. L'éco-épidémiologie - Vers une épidémiologie de la complexité [Eco-epidemiology: towards epidemiology of complexity]. Medical Science (Paris). 2016;**32**(5):500-505. French. DOI: 10.1051/medsci/20163205018

[13] Dubourg G, Raoult D, Fenollar F. Emerging methodologies for pathogen identification in bloodstream infections: An update. Expert Review of Molecular Diagnostics. 2019;**19**(2):161-173. DOI: 10.1080/14737159.2019.1568241

[14] Blauwkamp TA, Thair S, Rosen MJ, Blair L, Lindner MS, Vilfan ID, et al. Analytical and clinical validation of a microbial cell-free DNA sequencing test for infectious disease. Nature Microbiology. 2019;**4**(4):663-674. DOI: 10.1038/s41564-018-0349-6

[15] Miao Q, Ma Y, Wang Q, Pan J, Zhang Y, Jin W, et al. Microbiological diagnostic performance of metagenomic next-generation sequencing when applied to clinical practice. Clinical Infectious Diseases. 2018;**67**(suppl_2):S231-S240. DOI: 10.1093/cid/ciy693

[16] Wouters Y, Dalloyaux D, Christenhusz A, Roelofs HMJ, Wertheim HF, Bleeker-Rovers CP, et al. Droplet digital polymerase chain reaction for rapid broad-spectrum detection of bloodstream infections. Microbial Biotechnology. 2020;**13**(3):657-668. DOI: 10.1111/1751-7915.13491

[17] Simner PJ, Miller S, Carroll KC. Understanding the promises and hurdles of metagenomic next-generation sequencing as a diagnostic tool for infectious diseases. Clinical Infectious Diseases. 2018;**66**(5):778-788. DOI: 10.1093/cid/cix881

[18] Pomari E, Piubelli C, Perandin F, Bisoffi Z. Digital PCR: A new technology for diagnosis of parasitic infections. Clinical Microbiology and Infection. 2019;**25**(12):1510-1516. DOI: 10.1016/j.cmi.2019.06.009

[19] Watson JD, Crick FH. Molecular structure of nucleic acids; a structure for deoxyribose nucleic acid. Nature. 1953;**171**(4356):737-738. DOI: 10.1038/171737a0

[20] Maxam AM, Gilbert W. A new method for sequencing DNA. Proceedings of the National Academy of Sciences. 1977;**74**(2):560-564

[21] Sanger F, Coulson AR. A rapid method for determining sequences in DNA by primed synthesis with DNA polymerase. Journal of Molecular Biology. 1975;**94**:441-448. DOI: 10.1016/0022-2836(75)90213-2

[22] Hunkapiller M, Kent S, Caruthers M, Dreyer W, Firca J, Giffin C, et al. A microchemical facility for the analysis and synthesis of genes and proteins. Nature. 1984;**310**(5973):105-111. DOI: 10.1038/310105a0

[23] Smith LM, Sanders JZ, Kaiser RJ, Hughes P, Dodd C, Connell CR, et al. Fluorescence detection in automated DNA sequence analysis. Nature. 1986;**321**(6071):674-679. DOI: 10.1038/321674a0

[24] Hood LE, Hunkapiller MW, Smith LM. Automated DNA sequencing and analysis of the human genome. Genomics. 1987;**1**(3):201-212. DOI: 10.1016/0888-7543(87)90046-2

[25] Smith LM, Kaiser RJ, Sanders JZ, Hood LE. The synthesis and use of fluorescent oligonucleotides in DNA sequence analysis. Methods in Enzymology. 1987;**155**:260-301. DOI: 10.1016/0076-6879(87)55021-2

[26] McDonald LA, Kelley JM, Brandon RC, Adams MD. Optimization of applied Biosystems 373 sequencer stretch modification. BioTechniques. 1995;**19**(3):464-471

[27] Levy SE, Boone BE. Next-generation sequencing strategies. Cold Spring Harbor Perspectives in Medicine. 2019;**9**(7):a025791. DOI: 10.1101/cshperspect.a025791

[28] Margulies M, Egholm M, Altman WE, Attiya S, Bader JS, et al. Genome sequencing in microfabricated high-density picolitre reactors. Nature. 2005;**437**:376-380. DOI: 10.1038/nature03959

[29] Hernández M, Quijada NM, Rodríguez-Lázaro D, Eiros JM. Aplicación de la secuenciación masiva y la bioinformática al diagnóstico

microbiológico clínico [Bioinformatics of next generation sequencing in clinical microbiology diagnosis]. Revista Argentina de Microbiología. 2020;**52**(2):150-161. Spanish. DOI: 10.1016/j.ram.2019.06.003

[30] Slatko BE, Gardner AF, Ausubel FM. Overview of next-generation sequencing technologies. Current Protocols in Molecular Biology. 2018;**122**(1):e59. DOI: 10.1002/cpmb.59

[31] Kumar KR, Cowley MJ, Davis RL. Next-generation sequencing and emerging technologies. Seminars in Thrombosis and Hemostasis. 2019;**45**(7):661-673. DOI: 10.1055/s-0039-1688446

[32] Linnarsson S. Recent advances in DNA sequencing methods - general principles of sample preparation. Experimental Cell Research. 2010;**316**:1339-1343

[33] Garalde DR, Snell EA, Jachimowicz D, et al. Highly parallel direct RNA sequencing on an array of nanopores. Nature Methods. 2018;**15**(03):201-206

[34] Van der Auwera GA, Carneiro MO, Hartl C, et al. From FastQ data to high confidence variant calls: The genome analysis toolkit best practices pipeline. Current Protocols in Bioinformatics. 2013;**43**:1-33

[35] Pickrell WO, Rees MI, Chung SK. Next generation sequencing methodologies–an overview. Advances in Protein Chemistry and Structural Biology. 2012;**89**:1-26

[36] Hu T, Chitnis N, Monos D, Dinh A. Next-generation sequencing technologies: An overview. Human Immunology. 2021;**82**(11):801-811. DOI: 10.1016/j.humimm.2021.02.012

[37] Kleppe K, Ohtsuka E, Kleppe R, Molineux I, Khorana HG. Studies on polynucleotides. XCVI. Repair replications of short synthetic DNA's as catalyzed by DNA polymerases. Journal of Molecular Biology. 1971;**56**(2):341-361. DOI: 10.1016/0022-2836(71)90469-4

[38] Mullis K, Faloona F. Specific synthesis of DNA in vitro via a polymerase-catalyzed chain reaction. Methods in Enzymology. 1987;**155**:335-350

[39] Rappolee DA, Mark D, Banda MJ, Werb Z. Wound macrophages express TGF-alpha and other growth factors in vivo: Analysis by mRNA phenotyping. Science. 1988;**241**:708-712

[40] Gilliland G, Perrin S, Blanchard K, Bunn HF. Analysis of cytokine mRNA and DNA: Detection and quantitation by competitive polymerase chain reaction. Proceedings of the National Academy of Sciences of the United States of America. 1990;**87**:2725-2729

[41] Slomovic S, Schuster G. Circularized RT-PCR (cRT-PCR): Analysis of the 5′ ends, 3′ ends, and poly(a) tails of RNA. Methods in Enzymology. 2013;**530**:227-251. DOI: 10.1016/B978-0-12-420037-1.00013-0

[42] Triglia T, Peterson MG, Kemp DJ. A procedure for in vitro amplification of DNA segments that lie outside the boundaries of known sequences. Nucleic Acids Research. 1988;**16**(16):8186

[43] Dynon K, Varrasso A, Ficorilli N. Identification of equine herpesvirus 3 (equinecoital exanthema virus), equine gammaherpesviruses 2 and 5, equine adenoviruses 1 and 2, equine arteritis virus and equine rhinitis a virus by polymerase chain reaction. Australian Veterinary Journal. 2001;**79**:695-702

[44] Haase AT, Retzel EF, Staskus KA. Amplification and detection of lentiviral

DNA inside cells. Proceedings of the National Academy of Sciences of the United States of America. 1990;**87**(13):4971-4975. DOI: 10.1073/pnas.87.13.4971

[45] Chamberlain JS, Gibbs RA, Ranier JE, Nguyen PN, Caskey CT. Deletion screening of the Duchenne muscular dystrophy locus via multiplex DNA amplification. Nucleic Acids Research. 1988;**16**(23):11141-11156. DOI: 10.1093/nar/16.23.11141

[46] Hayden MJ, Nguyen TM, Waterman A, et al. Multiplex-ready PCR: A new method for multiplexed SSR and SNP genotyping. BMC Genomics. 2008;**9**:80. DOI: 10.1186/1471-2164-9-80

[47] Liu YG, Chen Y. High-efficiency thermal asymmetric interlaced PCR for amplification of unknown flanking sequences. BioTechniques. 2007;**43**(5):649-650, 652, 654 passim. DOI: 10.2144/000112601

[48] Troutt AB, McHeyzer-Williams MG, Pulendran B, Nossal GJ. Ligation-anchored PCR: A simple amplification technique with single-sided specificity. Proceedings of the National Academy of Sciences of the United States of America. 1992;**89**(20):9823-9825. DOI: 10.1073/pnas.89.20.9823

[49] Cheng S, Fockler C, Barnes WM, Higuchi R. Effective amplification of long targets from cloned inserts and human genomic DNA. Proceedings of the National Academy of Sciences of the United States of America. 1994;**91**(12):5695-5699

[50] Wittwer CT, Herrmann MG, Moss AA, Rasmussen RP. Continuous fluorescence monitoring of rapid cycle DNA amplification. BioTechniques. 1997;**22**(1):130-131, 134-8. DOI: 10.2144/97221bi01

[51] Chang LI-PCR. An ultrasensitive immunoassay for biomolecular detection. Analytical Chimica Acta. 2016;**910**:12-24

[52] Sykes PJ, Neoh SH, Brisco MJ, Hughes E, Condon J, Morley AA. Quantitation of targets for PCR by use of limiting dilution. BioTechniques. 1992;**13**(3):444-449

[53] Hindson BJ, Ness KD, Masquelier DA, Belgrader P, Heredia NJ, Makarewicz AJ, et al. High-throughput droplet digital PCR system for absolute quantitation of DNA copy number. Analytical Chemistry. 2011;**83**(22):8604-8610

[54] Notomi T, Okayama H, Masubuchi H, Yonekawa T, Watanabe K, Amino N, et al. Loop-mediated isothermal amplification of DNA. Nucleic Acids Research. 2000;**128**:E63

[55] Hardinge P, Murray JAH. Reduced false positives and improved reporting of loop-mediated isothermal amplification using quenched fluorescent primers. Scientific Reports. 2019;**9**:7400

[56] Rougemont M, Van Saanen M, Sahli R, Hinrikson HP, Bille J, Jaton K. Detection of four plasmodium species in blood from humans by 18S rRNA gene subunit-based and species-specific real-time PCR assays. Journal of Clinical Microbiology. 2004;**42**(12):5636-5643. DOI: 10.1128/JCM.42.12.5636-5643.2004

[57] Pohl G, IeM S. Principle and applications of digital PCR. Expert Review of Molecular Diagnostics. 2004;**4**(1):41-47. DOI: 10.1586/14737159.4.1.41

[58] Hall Sedlak R, Jerome KR. The potential advantages of digital PCR for clinical virology diagnostics. Expert Review of Molecular Diagnostics. 2014;**14**(4):501-507. DOI: 10.1586/14737159.2014.910456

[59] Belmonte FR, Martin JL, Frescura K, Damas J, Pereira F, Tarnopolsky MA, et al. Digital PCR methods improve detection sensitivity and measurement precision of low abundance mtDNA deletions. Scientific Reports. 2016;**6**:25186. DOI: 10.1038/srep25186

[60] Liu Z, Zhu L, Roberts R, Tong W. Toward clinical implementation of next-generation sequencing-based genetic testing in rare diseases: Where are we? Trends in Genetics. 2019;**35**:852-867. DOI: 10.1016/j.tig.2019.08.006

[61] Liu Z, Hatim Q, Thakkar S, Roberts R, Shi T. Editorial: Emerging technologies powering rare and neglected disease diagnosis and Theraphy development. Frontiers in Pharmacology. 2022;**13**:877401. DOI: 10.3389/fphar.2022.877401

[62] Carvalho KSS, da Silva Júnior WJ, da Silveira Regueira Neto M, Silva VC, de Sá Leitão Paiva Júnior S, Balbino VQ, et al. Application of next generation sequencing (NGS) for descriptive analysis of 30 genomes of Leishmania infantum isolates in middle-North Brazil. Scientific Reports. 2020;**10**(1):12321. DOI: 10.1038/s41598-020-68953-9

[63] Monteiro CC, Villegas LE, Campolina TB, Pires AC, Miranda JC, Pimenta PF, et al. Bacterial diversity of the American sand fly Lutzomyia intermedia using high-throughput metagenomic sequencing. Parasites & Vectors. 2016;**9**(1):480. DOI: 10.1186/s13071-016-1767-z

[64] Samaranayake N, Fernando SD, Neththikumara NF, Rodrigo C, Karunaweera ND, Dissanayake VH. Association of HLA class I and II genes with cutaneous leishmaniasis: A case control study from Sri Lanka and a systematic review. BMC Infectious Diseases. 2016;**16**:292. DOI: 10.1186/s12879-016-1626-8

[65] Ali RS, Newport MJ, Bakhiet SM, Ibrahim ME, Fahal AH. Host genetic susceptibility to mycetoma. PLoS Neglected Tropical Diseases. 2020;**14**(4):e0008053. DOI: 10.1371/journal.pntd.0008053

[66] Bourgard C, Albrecht L, Kayano ACAV, Sunnerhagen P, Costa FTM. Plasmodium vivax biology: Insights provided by genomics, transcriptomics and proteomics. Frontiers in Cellular and Infection Microbiology. 2018;**8**:34. DOI: 10.3389/fcimb.2018.00034

[67] Baptista RP, Reis-Cunha JL, DeBarry JD, Chiari E, Kissinger JC, Bartholomeu DC, et al. Assembly of highly repetitive genomes using short reads: The genome of discrete typing unit III Trypanosoma cruzi strain 231. Microbial Genomics. 2018;**4**(4):e000156. DOI: 10.1099/mgen.0.000156

[68] Gaur P, Chaturvedi A. Mining SNPs in extracellular vesicular transcriptome of Trypanosoma cruzi: A step closer to early diagnosis of neglected Chagas disease. PeerJ. 2016;**4**:e2693. DOI: 10.7717/peerj.2693

[69] Murillo-Solano C, Ramos-Ligonio A, López-Monteon A, Guzmán-Gómez D, Torres-Montero J, Herrera C, et al. Diversity of Trypanosoma cruzi parasites infecting Triatoma dimidiata in Central Veracruz, Mexico, and their one health ecological interactions. Infection, Genetics and Evolution. 2021;**95**:105050. DOI: 10.1016/j.meegid.2021.105050

[70] Strouhal M, Mikalová L, Haviernik J, Knauf S, Bruisten S, Noordhoek GT, et al. Complete genome sequences of two strains of Treponema pallidum subsp. pertenue from Indonesia: Modular structure of several treponemal genes. PLoS Neglected Tropical Diseases. 2018;**12**(10):e0006867. DOI: 10.1371/journal.pntd.0006867

[71] Delatorre E, Miranda M, Tschoeke DA, Carvalho de Sequeira P, Alves Sampaio S, Barbosa-Lima G, et al. An observational clinical case of Zika virus-associated neurological disease is associated with primary IgG response and enhanced TNF levels. The Journal of General Virology. 2018;**99**(7):913-916. DOI: 10.1099/jgv.0.001080

[72] Ko HY, Salem GM, Chang GJ, Chao DY. Application of next-generation sequencing to reveal how evolutionary dynamics of viral population shape dengue epidemiology. Frontiers in Microbiology. 2020;**11**:1371. DOI: 10.3389/fmicb.2020.01371

[73] Iamrod K, Chaidee A, Rucksaken R, Kopolrat KY, Worasith C, Wongphutorn P, et al. Development and efficacy of droplet digital PCR for detection of Strongyloides stercoralis in stool. The American Journal of Tropical Medicine and Hygiene. 2021;**106**(1):312-319. DOI: 10.4269/ajtmh.21-0729

[74] Ramírez JD, Herrera G, Hernández C, Cruz-Saavedra L, Muñoz M, Flórez C, et al. Evaluation of the analytical and diagnostic performance of a digital droplet polymerase chain reaction (ddPCR) assay to detect Trypanosoma cruzi DNA in blood samples. PLoS Neglected Tropical Diseases. 2018;**12**(12):e0007063. DOI: 10.1371/journal.pntd.0007063

[75] Mairiang D, Songjaeng A, Hansuealueang P, Malila Y, Lertsethtakarn P, Silapong S, et al. Application of one-step reverse transcription droplet digital PCR for dengue virus detection and quantification in clinical specimens. Diagnostics (Basel). 2021;**11**(4):639. DOI: 10.3390/diagnostics11040639

[76] Navarro Sanchez ME, Devard N, Houy C, Abachin E, Godard S, Esson R, et al. Multiplex reverse transcriptase droplet digital PCR for the simultaneous quantification of four dengue serotypes: Proof of concept study. Biologicals. 2020;**67**:62-68. DOI: 10.1016/j.biologicals.2020.06.001

[77] Koepfli C, Nguitragool W, Hofmann NE, Robinson LJ, Ome-Kaius M, Sattabongkot J, et al. Sensitive and accurate quantification of human malaria parasites using droplet digital PCR (ddPCR). Scientific Reports. 2016;**6**:39183. DOI: 10.1038/srep39183

[78] Hu B, Tao Y, Shao Z, Zheng Y, Zhang R, Yang X, et al. A comparison of blood pathogen detection among droplet digital PCR, metagenomic next-generation sequencing, and blood culture in critically ill patients with suspected bloodstream infections. Frontiers in Microbiology. 2021;**12**:641202. DOI: 10.3389/fmicb.2021.641202

[79] Pilotte N, Maasch JRMA, Easton AV, Dahlstrom E, Nutman TB, Williams SA. Targeting a highly repeated germline DNA sequence for improved real-time PCR-based detection of Ascaris infection in human stool. PLoS Neglected Tropical Diseases. 2019;**13**(7):e0007593. DOI: 10.1371/journal.pntd.0007593

[80] Chen B, Chen Z, Yang YS, Cai GL, Xu XJ, Guan HZ, et al. Next-generation sequencing combined with serological tests based pathogen analysis for a neurocysticercosis patient with a 20-year history:A case report. BMC Neurology. 2021;**21**(1):236. DOI: 10.1186/s12883-021-02277-7

[81] Fei X, Li C, Zhang Y, Zhang H, Liu X, Ji X, et al. Data relating to sequencing statistics and the reads and genomic coverage aligning to Taenia solium in the cerebrospinal fluid. Data in Brief. 2020;**31**:105700. DOI: 10.1016/j.dib.2020.105700

[82] Pajuelo MJ, Eguiluz M, Dahlstrom E, Requena D, Guzmán F, Ramirez M, et al. Cysticercosis working Group in Peru. Identification and characterization of microsatellite markers derived from the whole genome analysis of Taenia solium. PLoS Neglected Tropical Diseases. 2015;**9**(12):e0004316. DOI: 10.1371/journal.pntd.0004316

[83] Maganira JD, Kidima W, Mwita CJ, Halvarsson P, Höglund J. Soil contamination by Taenia solium egg DNA in rural villages in Kongwa district, Tanzania. Infection Ecology & Epidemiology. 2020;**10**(1):1772668. DOI: 10.1080/20008686.2020.1772668

[84] Maganira JD, Mwang'onde BJ, Kidima W, Mwita CJ, Nkwengulila G, Höglund J. Validation of droplet digital polymerase chain reaction for the detection and absolute quantification of Taenia solium eggs in spiked soil samples. Acta Tropica. 2019;**200**:105175. DOI: 10.1016/j.actatropica.2019.105175

[85] Patiño LH, Castillo-Castañeda AC, Muñoz M, Jaimes JE, Luna-Niño N, Hernández C, et al. Development of an amplicon-based next-generation sequencing protocol to identify Leishmania species and other Trypanosomatids in Leishmaniasis endemic areas. Microbiology Spectrum. 2021;**9**(2):e0065221. DOI: 10.1128/Spectrum.00652-21

[86] Kamath K, Reifert J, Johnston T, Gable C, Pantazes RJ, Rivera HN, et al. Antibody epitope repertoire analysis enables rapid antigen discovery and multiplex serology. Scientific Reports. 2020;**10**(1):5294. DOI: 10.1038/s41598-020-62256-9

[87] Camacho E, Rastrojo A, Sanchiz Á, González-de la Fuente S, Aguado B, Requena JM. Leishmania mitochondrial genomes: Maxicircle structure and heterogeneity of Minicircles. Genes (Basel). 2019;**10**(10):758. DOI: 10.3390/genes10100758

[88] Mukherjee A, Boisvert S, Monte-Neto RL, Coelho AC, Raymond F, Mukhopadhyay R, et al. Telomeric gene deletion and intrachromosomal amplification in antimony-resistant Leishmania. Molecular Microbiology. 2013;**88**(1):189-202. DOI: 10.1111/mmi.12178

[89] Muxel SM, Aoki JI, Fernandes JCR, Laranjeira-Silva MF, Zampieri RA, Acuña SM, et al. Arginine and polyamines fate in Leishmania infection. Frontiers in Microbiology. 2018;**8**:2682. DOI: 10.3389/fmicb.2017.02682

[90] Ramírez JD, Herrera G, Muskus C, Mendez C, Duque MC, Butcher R. Development of a digital droplet polymerase chain reaction (ddPCR) assay to detect Leishmania DNA in samples from cutaneous Leishmaniasis patients. International Journal of Infectious Diseases. 2019;**79**:1-3. DOI: 10.1016/j.ijid.2018.10.029

[91] Fan Y, Chen J, Liu M, Xu X, Zhang Y, Yue P, et al. Application of droplet digital PCR to detection of mycobacterium tuberculosis and mycobacterium leprae infections: A narrative review. Infection and Drug Resistance. 2022;**15**:1067-1076. DOI: 10.2147/IDR.S349607

[92] Cheng X, Sun L, Zhao Q, Mi Z, Yu G, Wang Z, et al. Development and evaluation of a droplet digital PCR assay for the diagnosis of paucibacillary leprosy in skin biopsy specimens. PLoS Neglected Tropical Diseases. 2019;**13**(3):e0007284. DOI: 10.1371/journal.pntd.0007284

[93] Wang D, Fan Y, Malhi M, Bi R, Wu Y, Xu M, et al. Missense variants in HIF1A and LACC1 contribute to leprosy risk

in Han Chinese. American Journal of Human Genetics. 2018;**102**(5):794-805. DOI: 10.1016/j.ajhg.2018.03.006

[94] Schachter J. Will droplet digital PCR become the test of choice for detecting and quantifying ocular chlamydia trachomatis infection? Maybe not. Expert Review of Molecular Diagnostics. 2013;**13**(8):789-792. DOI: 10.1586/14737159.2013.847792

[95] Roberts CH, Last A, Molina-Gonzalez S, Cassama E, Butcher R, Nabicassa M, et al. Development and evaluation of a next-generation digital PCR diagnostic assay for ocular chlamydia trachomatis infections. Journal of Clinical Microbiology. 2013;**51**(7):2195-2203. DOI: 10.1128/JCM.00622-13

[96] Thurlow CM, Joseph SJ, Ganova-Raeva L, Katz SS, Pereira L, Chen C, et al. Selective whole-genome amplification as a tool to enrich specimens with low Treponema pallidum genomic DNA copies for whole-genome sequencing. mSphere. 2022;**7**(3):e0000922. DOI: 10.1128/msphere.00009-22

[97] Seitz A, Hanssen F, Nieselt K. DACCOR-detection, characterization, and reconstruction of repetitive regions in bacterial genomes. PeerJ. 2018;**6**:e4742. DOI: 10.7717/peerj.4742

[98] Sun J, Meng Z, Wu K, Liu B, Zhang S, Liu Y, et al. Tracing the origin of Treponema pallidum in China using next-generation sequencing. Oncotarget. 2016;**7**(28):42904-42918. DOI: 10.18632/oncotarget.10154

[99] Romeis E, Tantalo L, Lieberman N, Phung Q, Greninger A, Giacani L. Genetic engineering of Treponema pallidum subsp. pallidum, the syphilis spirochete. PLoS Pathogens. 2021;**17**(7):e1009612. DOI: 10.1371/journal.ppat.1009612

[100] Calvelage S, Freuling CM, Fooks AR, Höper D, Marston DA, McElhinney L, et al. Full-genome sequences and phylogenetic analysis of archived Danish European bat lyssavirus 1 (EBLV-1) emphasize a higher genetic resolution and spatial segregation for sublineage 1a. Viruses. 2021;**13**(4):634. DOI: 10.3390/v13040634

[101] Calvelage S, Tammiranta N, Nokireki T, Gadd T, Eggerbauer E, Zaeck LM, et al. Genetic and Antigenetic characterization of the novel Kotalahti bat lyssavirus (KBLV). Viruses. 2021;**13**(1):69. DOI: 10.3390/v13010069

[102] Sanhueza D, Guégan JF, Jordan H, Chevillon C. Environmental variations in mycobacterium ulcerans transcriptome: Absence of Mycolactone expression in suboptimal environments. Toxins (Basel). 2019;**11**(3):146. DOI: 10.3390/toxins11030146

[103] Eddyani M, Vandelannoote K, Meehan CJ, Bhuju S, Porter JL, Aguiar J, et al. A genomic approach to resolving relapse versus reinfection among four cases of Buruli ulcer. PLoS Neglected Tropical Diseases. 2015;**9**(11):e0004158. DOI: 10.1371/journal.pntd.0004158

[104] Yu Z, Zhao Z, Chen L, Li J, Ju X. Development of a droplet digital PCR for detection of Trichuriasis in sheep. The Journal of Parasitology. 2020;**106**(5):603-610. DOI: 10.1645/20-16

[105] Armoo S, Doyle SR, Osei-Atweneboana MY, Grant WN. Significant heterogeneity in Wolbachia copy number within and between populations of Onchocerca volvulus. Parasites & Vectors. 2017;**10**(1):188. DOI: 10.1186/s13071-017-2126-4

[106] Zulch MF, Pilotte N, Grant JR, Minetti C, Reimer LJ, Williams SA. Selection and exploitation of prevalent, tandemly repeated genomic targets for improved real-time PCR-based detection of Wuchereria bancrofti and plasmodium falciparum in mosquitoes. PLoS One. 2020;**15**(5):e0232325. DOI: 10.1371/journal.pone.0232325

[107] Jongthawin J, Intapan PM, Lulitanond V, Sanpool O, Thanchomnang T, Sadaow L, et al. Detection and quantification of Wuchereria bancrofti and Brugia malayi DNA in blood samples and mosquitoes using duplex droplet digital polymerase chain reaction. Parasitology Research. 2016;**115**(8):2967-2972. DOI: 10.1007/s00436-016-5051-0

[108] Michalski ML, Weil GJ. Gender-specific gene expression in Brugia malayi. Molecular and Biochemical Parasitology. 1999;**104**(2):247-257. DOI: 10.1016/s0166-6851(99)00149-8

[109] Haçarız O, Akgün M, Kavak P, Yüksel B, Sağıroğlu MŞ. Comparative transcriptome profiling approach to glean virulence and immunomodulation-related genes of Fasciola hepatica. BMC Genomics. 2015;**16**(1):366. DOI: 10.1186/s12864-015-1539-8

[110] Biswal DK, Ghatani S, Shylla JA, Sahu R, Mullapudi N, Bhattacharya A, et al. An integrated pipeline for next generation sequencing and annotation of the complete mitochondrial genome of the giant intestinal fluke, Fasciolopsis buski (Lankester, 1857) Looss, 1899. PeerJ. 2013;**1**:e207. DOI: 10.7717/peerj.207

[111] Almeida LV, Coqueiro-Dos-Santos A, Rodriguez-Luiz GF, McCulloch R, Bartholomeu DC, Reis-Cunha JL. Chromosomal copy number variation analysis by next generation sequencing confirms ploidy stability in Trypanosoma brucei subspecies. Microbial Genomics. 2018;**4**(10):e000223. DOI: 10.1099/mgen.0.000223

[112] Jerome H, Taylor C, Sreenu VB, Klymenko T, Filipe A, Jackson C, et al. Metagenomic next-generation sequencing aids the diagnosis of viral infections in febrile returning travellers. The Journal of Infection. 2019;**79**(4):383-388. DOI: 10.1016/j.jinf.2019.08.003

[113] Almeida PR, Eisen AKA, Demoliner M, Spilki FR. RT-dPCR in mosquito samples for ZIKV detection: Effects of RNA extraction and reverse transcription in target concentration. Viruses. 2020;**12**(8):827. DOI: 10.3390/v12080827

[114] Saha S, Ramesh A, Kalantar K, Malaker R, Hasanuzzaman M, Khan LM, et al. Unbiased metagenomic sequencing for pediatric meningitis in Bangladesh reveals Neuroinvasive chikungunya virus outbreak and other unrealized pathogens. MBio. 2019;**10**(6):e02877-e02819. DOI: 10.1128/mBio.02877-19

[115] Bohl JA, Lay S, Chea S, Ahyong V, Parker DM, Gallagher S, et al. Discovering disease-causing pathogens in resource-scarce Southeast Asia using a global metagenomic pathogen monitoring system. Proceedings of the National Academy of Sciences of the United States of America. 2022;**119**(11):e2115285119. DOI: 10.1073/pnas.2115285119

[116] Cole DC, Crissman CC, Orozco AF. Canada's International Development Research Centre's eco-health projects with Latin Americans: Origins, development and challenges. Canadian Journal of Public Health. 2006;**97**(6):I8-I14

[117] Waltner-Toews D. Eco-health: A primer for veterinarians. The Canadian Veterinary Journal. 2009;**50**(5):519-521

[118] Díaz C, Torres Y, Cruz AM, Álvarez AM, Piquero ME, Valero AF. Estrategia intersectorial y participativa con enfoque de ecosalud para la prevención de la transmisión de dengue en el nivel local. Cadernos de Saúde Pública. 2009;**25**(Supl 1):S59-S70. DOI: 10.1590/S0102-311X2009001300006

[119] Mertens F, Saint-Charles J, Mergler D, Passos CJ, Lucotte M. Network approach for analyzing and promoting equity in participatory Ecohealth research. EcoHealth. 2005;**2**(2):113-126. DOI: 10.1007/s10393-004-0162-y

[120] Charron FD. Ecohealth Research in Practice: Innovative Applications of an Ecosystem Approach to Health. Ottawa, Canada: Springer/IDRC; 2012

[121] Wu Z, Lu L, Du J, Yang L, Ren X, Liu B, et al. Comparative analysis of rodent and small mammal viromes to better understand the wildlife origin of emerging infectious diseases. Microbiome. 2018;**6**(1):178. DOI: 10.1186/s40168-018-0554-9

[122] Faleye TOC, George UE, Klapsa D, Majumdar M, Oragwa AO, Adewumi MO, et al. Isolation and genomic characterization of echovirus 11 from faeces of a non-human primate in Nigeria. EcoHealth. 2020;**17**(4):461-468. DOI: 10.1007/s10393-021-01515-1

[123] Giraldo LM, Muñoz M, Hernández C, Herrera G, Velásquez-Ortiz N, Cantillo-Barraza O, et al. Identification of blood-feeding sources in Panstrongylus, Psammolestes, Rhodnius and Triatoma using amplicon-based next-generation sequencing. Parasites & Vectors. 2020;**13**(1):434. DOI: 10.1186/s13071-020-04310-z

[124] Dumonteil E, Ramirez-Sierra MJ, Pérez-Carrillo S, Teh-Poot C, Herrera C, Gourbière S, et al. Detailed ecological associations of triatomines revealed by metabarcoding and next-generation sequencing: Implications for triatomine behavior and Trypanosoma cruzi transmission cycles. Scientific Reports. 2018;**8**(1):4140. DOI: 10.1038/s41598-018-22455-x

[125] Pronovost H, Peterson AC, Chavez BG, Blum MJ, Dumonteil E, Herrera CP. Deep sequencing reveals multiclonality and new discrete typing units of Trypanosoma cruzi in rodents from the southern United States. Journal of Microbiology, Immunology, and Infection. 2020;**53**(4):622-633. DOI: 10.1016/j.jmii.2018.12.004

[126] Li H, Bai R, Zhao Z, Tao L, Ma M, Ji Z, et al. Application of droplet digital PCR to detect the pathogens of infectious diseases. Bioscience Reports. 2018;**38**(6):BSR20181170. DOI: 10.1042/BSR20181170

[127] Chen B, Jiang Y, Cao X, Liu C, Zhang N, Shi D. Droplet digital PCR as an emerging tool in detecting pathogens nucleic acids in infectious diseases. Clinica Chimica Acta. 2021;**517**:156-161. DOI: 10.1016/j.cca.2021.02.008

[128] Rang FJ, Kloosterman WP, de Ridder J. From squiggle to basepair: Computational approaches for improving nanopore sequencing read accuracy. Genome Biology. 2018;**19**(1):90. DOI: 10.1186/s13059-018-1462-9

[129] Ari S, Arikan M. Next-generation sequencing: Advantages, disadvantages, and future. In: Hakeem KR, Tombuloğlu H, Tombuloğlu G, editors. Plant Omics: Trends and Applications. Switzerland: Springer International Publishing; 2016. DOI: 10.1007/978-3-319-31703-8_5

[130] Wenger AM, Peluso P, Rowell WJ, Chang PC, Hall RJ, Concepcion GT, et al. Accurate circular consensus long-read sequencing improves variant detection and assembly of a human genome. Nature Biotechnology. 2019;**37**(10):1155-1162. DOI: 10.1038/s41587-019-0217-9

[131] Charalampous T, Richardson H, Kay GL, Baldan R, Jeanes C, Rae D, et al. Rapid diagnosis of lower respiratory infection using nanopore-based clinical metagenomics. bioRxiv. 2018:387548 [Preprint]

[132] Couto N, Schuele L, Raangs EC, Machado MP, Mendes CI, Jesus TF, et al. Author correction: Critical steps in clinical shotgun metagenomics for the concomitant detection and typing of microbial pathogens. Scientific Reports. 2019;**9**(1):6406. DOI: 10.1038/s41598-019-42134-9

[133] Deurenberg RH, Bathoorn E, Chlebowicz MA, Couto N, Ferdous M, García-Cobos S, et al. Application of next generation sequencing in clinical microbiology and infection prevention. Journal of Biotechnology. 2017;**243**:16-24. DOI: 10.1016/j.jbiotec.2016.12.022

[134] Rohit A, Suresh Kumar D, Dhinakaran I, Joy J, Vijay Kumar D, Kumar Ballamoole K, et al. Whole-genome-based analysis reveals multiclone Serratia marcescens outbreaks in a non-neonatal intensive care unit setting in a tertiary care hospital in India. Journal of Medical Microbiology. 2019;**68**(4):616-621. DOI: 10.1099/jmm.0.000947

[135] Roy S, Hartley J, Dunn H, Williams R, Williams CA, Breuer J. Whole-genome sequencing provides data for stratifying infection prevention and control Management of Nosocomial Influenza a. Clinical Infectious Diseases. 2019;**69**(10):1649-1656. DOI: 10.1093/cid/ciz020

[136] Costa DM, Johani K, Melo DS, Lopes LKO, Lopes Lima LKO, Tipple AFV, et al. Biofilm contamination of high-touched surfaces in intensive care units: Epidemiology and potential impacts. Letters in Applied Microbiology. 2019;**68**(4):269-276. DOI: 10.1111/lam.13127

[137] Wilson M, Glaser KC, Adams-Fish D, Boley M, Mayda M, Molestina RE. Development of droplet digital PCR for the detection of Babesia microti and Babesia duncani. Experimental Parasitology. 2015;**149**:24e31. DOI: 10.1016/j.exppara.2014.12.003

Chapter 2

Vector Control: Insights Arising from the Post-Genomics Findings on Insects' Reproductive Biology

Isabela Ramos and Fabio Gomes

Abstract

The high prevalence of neglected vector-borne diseases, such as Chagas disease and dengue fever, imposes enormous health and financial burdens in developing countries. Historically, and still, to this day, the main effective methods to manage those diseases rely on vector population control. Although early efforts in understanding vector-specific biology resulted in important advancements in the development of strategies for the management of vector-borne diseases, studies regarding the complex physiology of local vector species were weakened by the expanding use of insecticide-based tools, which were, at the time, proven simpler and effective. The rising threat of insecticide resistance and climate change (which can expand endemic areas) has reemphasized the need to rely on thorough species-specific vector biology. One approach to controlling vector populations is to disrupt molecular processes or antagonize the metabolic targets required to produce viable eggs. Here, we discuss new findings arising from post-genomics molecular studies on vector reproductive biology and discuss their potential for the elaboration of new effective vector control interventions.

Keywords: reproductive biology, post-genomics, evidence-based vector control

1. Introduction

1.1 Vector-borne diseases

Vector-borne diseases remain among the deadliest and most prevalent infectious diseases worldwide. Mosquito-transmitted arboviral diseases inflict an enormous burden in tropical areas of the world. A previous study estimated that almost 400 million people are infected by the dengue virus (DENV) every year [1]. While tremendous progress on vector control has been made over the twentieth and twenty-first centuries, we are now facing a critical moment. Record-breaking numbers of dengue cases were detected in the Americas in 2019 [2]. This is aggravated by the fact that multiple serotypes circulate in these regions, maximizing the risk of hemorrhagic fever and other severe complications. Other arboviruses are also of concern. For example, the Zika virus (ZIKV), transmitted by *Aedes aegypti*, rapidly spread in the Americas in 2014–2015, where it was linked with a surge of newborn malformations, including microcephaly [3, 4], inflicting a lifelong impact on children, their parents, and the health public system. Other viruses, like Mayaro (MAYV), chikungunya (CHKV), and yellow fever (YFV), continue to circulate and periodically reemerge. In addition to the arboviruses, vector-borne parasitic diseases, such as Chagas disease, are also medically important. The triatomine bug *Rhodnius prolixus* is a primary vector of *Trypanosoma cruzi*, the causative agent of Chagas disease, a neglected disease endemic to Central and South America. Chagas disease remains the main cause of death related to neglected infectious diseases in the Americas. Currently, Chagas affects approximately 8 million people and migration among endemic and non-endemic regions has expanded its occurrence to approximately 350,000 infected carriers around the globe [5].

Overall, these diseases not only result in a high number of deaths and hospitalizations but also generate a huge economic impact due to the disability of people during their learning and working ages [6, 7]. While most restricted to tropical areas, where vectors meet the perfect conditions for mating and reproduction, models of climate change predict an expansion of the global areas suitable for vector reproduction. Under these models, areas of Europe and America have already seen an increase in the suitability of vector populations and this trend is going to accelerate in the following decades [8, 9]. This is of special concern as these pathogens meet an immunologically naive local population lacking any previous exposure to such diseases.

2. Reproduction as a target for vector control

The interference in insect vector natural populations has remained one of the key strategies for the control of vector-borne diseases. For the past 50 years, vector control policies have relied on the utilization of insecticide-based tools. With the rising of resistance spreading across populations, a major threat to the ongoing success of control programs has been acknowledged [10].

Although insects are the largest and most diverse group of animals on the planet, most species are regarded as species with a high reproductive capacity. Females can generally produce a large number of eggs in a short period, and the high rates of embryo viability boost their natural populations. Blood-feeding (hematophagy) is necessary for most human disease vectors to obtain the energy and nutrients required for efficient oogenesis, enabling the abovementioned high rates of oviposition [11]. Within a vector reproductive cycle, the overall process of converting protein from the blood meal into yolk protein precursors (YPPs), as well as coordinating their delivery to developing oocytes is the most complex stage of reproduction and requires the coordination of intricate metabolic and neuroendocrine pathways in the adult female. As a result, a comprehensive understanding of the complexity of egg production is the most promising approach to designing safe tools for interference in vector reproduction (**Figure 1**).

The molecular physiology of oogenesis is highly conserved within the different insect vectors [11–13]. In brief, oogenesis is triggered by signals from nutritional status and the blood meal. The levels of the sesquiterpene juvenile hormone (JH) [14], secreted by the *corpora allata* in the brain, increase over the early periods of insect maturity triggering changes in the fat body that become sensitive to the ovary-producing steroid hormone ecdysone [15]. After the blood meal, the brain stops JH synthesis and releases the ovarian ecdysiotropic hormone, signaling to the ovaries to produce ecdysone. In the fat body, ecdysone is hydroxylated to 20-hydroxyecdysone

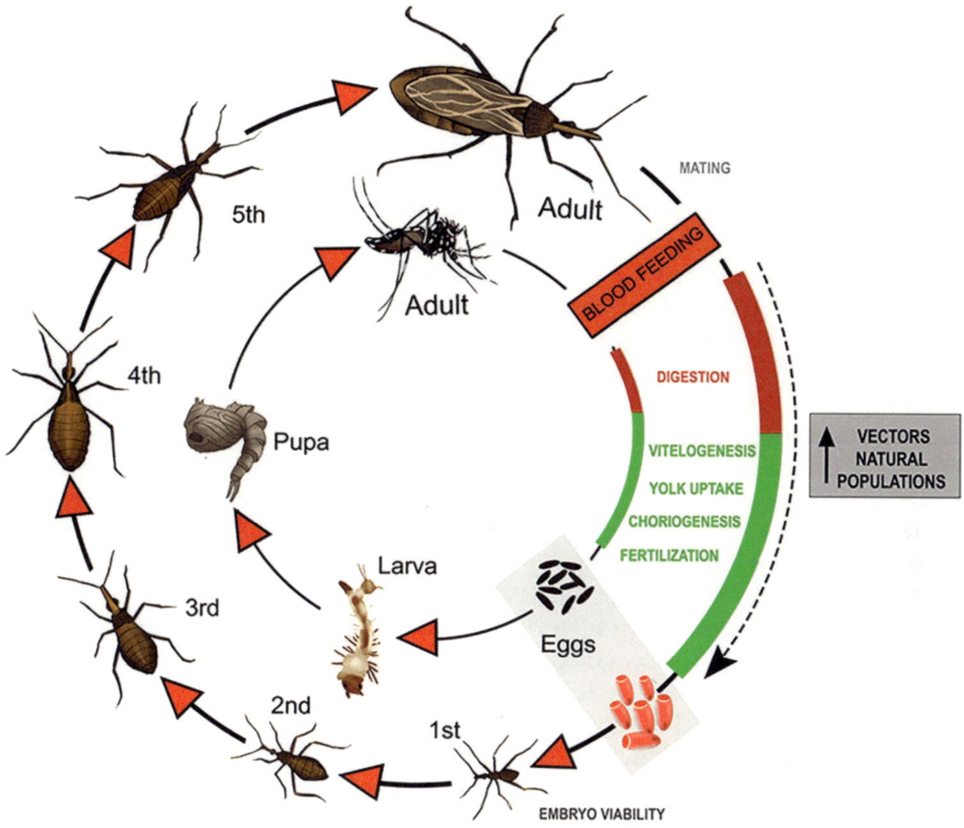

Figure 1.
Targets for intervention within the reproductive cycle of vectors. After digestion, adult females are able to lay a large number of highly viable eggs, thus contributing to the increase and maintenance of vector natural populations. The complex physiology process of transforming the contents of the blood meal into mature fertilized eggs requires intricate coordination to accomplish vitellogenesis, delivery of the yolk to the oocytes (yolk uptake), eggshell biogenesis (choriogenesis), and fertilization (mating habits). Interference in any of those stages directly impairs vectors' egg production capacity and embryo viability, rendering drastically reduced reproduction rates.

(20E) and binds to the 20E receptor EcR/USP to trigger vitellogenesis, that is, the production of the YPPs (yolk protein precursors). YPPs are secreted to the hemolymph and delivered to the developing oocytes in the ovaries via receptor-mediated endocytosis. Apart from the huge metabolic challenge of transforming the blood meal into a large number of eggs, the maximum capacity of egg production is also dependent on successful mating, fertilization, and proper conditions for embryo development [12, 16–23].

3. Potential targets for intervention within vectors reproduction

3.1 The molecular mechanisms of vitellogenesis and oogenesis

The conversion of protein from the blood meal into YPPs for eggs biogenesis is a vital component of the reproductive cycle and understanding how this process is regulated is necessary to design safe, specific, and effective ways to block reproduction in vectors. Mosquito 20E has been shown to play multiple roles in *Anopheles.*

Apart from regulating monogamy in *Anopheles*, the male-transferred 20E was shown to be important in maintaining sperm viability over the female lifetime through induction of the heme peroxidase 15 (HPX15) [24]. Accordingly, HPX15 knockdown was shown to dramatically increase the ratio of infertile eggs. Upon insemination, the male 20E further interacts with the female Mating-Induced Stimulator of Oogenesis (MISO) and induces an increase in fecundity by increasing the expression of LP and oocyte numbers [25]. Finally, 20E was also shown to be necessary for *Anopheles* egg-laying [26].

On that note, several genes that are somehow essential for oogenesis and generate unviable embryos have been identified and functionally tested in *R. prolixus.* The orthologue of Bicaudal C (*Bic*C), a gene originally identified in *D. melanogaster* involved in embryonic patterning has shown to be maternally expressed and essential for the arrangement of the follicle cells [27]. The control of iron and heme homeostasis is particularly critical for hematophagous insects, especially for the strictly hematophagous triatomines, such *R. prolixus*. In this model, the silencing of multiple iron-related genes, namely, ferritin, iron responsive protein 1 (IRP1), heme oxygenase (HO), and heme exporter feline leukemia virus C receptor (FLVCR), impairs oogenesis and embryo viability [28, 29].

The role of receptor-mediated endocytosis in yolk uptake has been investigated in oocytes of many insect species. The internalization of yolk proteins through the presence of a specialized endocytic cortex in the oocytes, which includes prominent microvilli, coated pits, coated vesicles, and endosomes have been shown in several species, including *Aedes* [30–38] However, the regulations encompassing the recruitment of the endocytic machinery to specific sites of the oocyte cortex and the signals that govern the oocyte endocytic pathways and endosomal maturation are yet to be addressed. In *R. prolixus*, ATG6/Beclin1 class-III PI3K complexes I and II were shown to be essential for YPP uptake. Insects silenced for the genes present in both complexes produce yolk-deficient eggs generating unviable embryos due to the lack of generated phosphatidylinositol-3P (PI3P) to recruit the endocytic machinery in vitellogenic oocytes [39, 40].

3.2 Choriogenesis as an emerging target for safe interventions

The final checkpoint of oogenesis, before fertilization, is the triggering of the choriogenesis program, in which the multiple layers of the chorion are secreted by the follicle cells that envelop the developing oocytes. Remarkably, while the chorion's primary protective function is conserved in insects, its general composition and structure have evolved in a highly species-specific manner, giving rise to a wide range of morphologies and functional adaptations. The main chorion proteins in insects have been identified in models, such as the silk moth *Bombyx mori*, the fruit fly *D. melanogaster,* and the mosquito *Aedes Aegypti*, and revealed to be broadly unrelated to their counterparts in each of these species [41, 42]. Proteins that are conserved in a wide variety of organisms are not ideal target molecules as vector control agents because of deleterious effects on non-target organisms, such as vertebrates, pollinating agricultural insects, and beneficial predators. As a result, studies on the molecular biology of the chorion biogenesis in insect vectors are biotechnology strategic as they are likely to unravel safe molecular targets that are at the same time essential for reproduction and highly specific to one species.

The *A. aegypti* eggshell is composed of different structural proteins, enzymes, odorant-binding proteins, as well as many uncharacterized proteins of unknown function. Melanization proteins and enzymes of the eggshell have been identified [43–49], and proteomics studies have been performed [42]. Isoe and colleagues [50] designed *in silico* analyses to identify mosquito-specific genes that are essential for successful embryo development. After systematic RNAi functional screening of over 40 selected genes, the authors identified a chorion-related protein named eggshell organizing factor 1 (EOF1), which is essential for eggshell biogenesis and embryo development. The EOF1 sequence includes an F-box functional motif, which is characterized by the interaction with the SKP1 protein in the SCF E3 ubiquitin ligase complex [51]. Although its exact function in the eggshell has not been elucidated, such findings are very promising in terms of designing safe strategies for vector control.

In *R. prolixus*, some aspects of the chorion ultrastructure and permeability properties were previously explored [52–54] and the identification of the specific chorion proteins Rp30 and Rp45, the latter associated with antifungal activity, was also described [55]. In this model, the cell biology of the follicle cells (FCs), the tissue that synthesizes and secretes the chorion components, has been explored. Early transcriptome analysis showed that the FCs are committed to transcription, translation, and vesicular traffic [56]. Accordingly, electron microscopy evidenced the FC's typical secretory cell morphology with a high content of vesiculated rough endoplasmic reticulum [57, 58]. Systemic RNAi experiments targeting the autophagy-related genes ULK1/ATG1, the autophagy-dedicated E2-conjugating enzyme ATG3 [57, 59], and E1-activating and E2-conjugating ubiquitin enzymes [60] generated particular phenotypes of chorion malformations due to alterations in the general protein homeostasis of the FCs during choriogenesis, resulting in extremely lower rates of embryo viability. Taken together, the data points to a high degree of complexity in the chorion biogenesis program in *R. prolixus*, rendering the process extremely sensitive to changes in proteostasis of the FCs, and, thus, an interesting target for slight but effective interventions.

Resistance to desiccation is another potential intervention target. Although mosquito eggs are laid in water, they are susceptible to dehydration in the first hours of development. Thus, this property directly affects mosquito reproduction. In *A. Aegypti*, the serosal cuticle secretion (an inner layer of the chorion secreted during embryogenesis) coincides with an increase in dry resistance and the presence of chitin as one of the serosal cuticle components has been detected [61–63]. In *R. prolixus*, chitin was detected in the ovaries and the embryonic cuticle [64, 65]. Additionally, exposure to lufenuron (a chitin synthesis inhibitor) and chitin synthase RNAi experiments reduced oviposition and embryo viability [66]. Therefore, the synthesis and deposition of chitin or chitin-like components in the eggshells are also promising targets for reproduction interventions.

Altogether, and combined with the above-mentioned high degree of species-specificity of the chorion proteins, choriogenesis has the potential to emerge as the foremost target for the generation of new and environmentally safe strategies to achieve vector control.

3.3 Molecular neuroendocrine control of egg production

Major advancements have been achieved in the understanding of the neurohormonal control of egg production. In *R. prolixus*, a detailed model depicting the control of oogenesis, ovulation, and oviposition has been designed and elegantly reviewed by Lange and colleagues [13]. Post-genomics has allowed the identification and functional characterization of dozens of reproduction-related neuropeptide receptor families, processing enzymes, and neurochemicals. Historically, *R. prolixus* has been an important model, wherein the basics of insect physiology have been determined [67–70]. Interestingly, the integration of the post-genomics findings with the smartly designed early physiology experiments has allowed the elucidation and depiction of many aspects of the global endocrinal integration in this vector.

3.4 Crosstalk between reproduction and immunity

A relationship between reproductive potential and immune status has been long established. Collectively, these studies suggest a tradeoff between immune activation and egg production, reflected by the identification of follicular atresia and other cell death pathways [71, 72]. Recent advances are now highlighting the role of nutrient-sensing pathways and vector immunometabolism [73]. Future studies will provide further insight into how signaling pathways, such as TOR and Insulin pathways, well-known vitellogenic and immune regulators, coordinate energetic balance during infection. Interestingly, previous work using natural combinations of vector-parasite has suggested that coevolution might have minimized the impact of infection [74], possibly by the fact that immune tolerance can induce a less-energetic costly immune response.

Rerouting of yolk components can be used as a nutritional factor for parasite development. Mosquito LP has been incorporated into *Plasmodium* oocyst as a lipid source [75]. While parasite development was accelerated by LP delivery, it did not induce any detectable reproductive cost [76]. Interestingly, mosquito lipids influenced not only total parasite numbers, but also *Plasmodium* sporozoite virulence upon transmission to vertebrate hosts [77]. Similarly, VG is a key component for *Plasmodium* survival. An interplay between YPPs and immune response has been demonstrated. Both LP and VG were shown to reduce the efficiency of the binding of the major parasite-killing TEP1 [78], increasing parasite survival following mosquito infection.

3.5 Interventions on mosquito mating and insemination

Mosquitoes are thought to use a set of sonorous, visual, and chemical cues to identify and attract their partners. While the manipulation of such signals used to guide mosquitoes is an interesting target to prevent mosquito mating, the molecular identity of its components, such as sex pheromones and their odorant-binding receptors are scant. In that sense, both *Anopheles* and *Aedes* mosquitoes can adopt a swarming behavior during mating. Aggregation pheromones have been identified in *Anopheles* [79]. Such compounds can be used to manipulate mating behavior in wild vector populations and are a likely target of vector control strategies. More recently, genes regulating cuticular hydrocarbon productions and the circadian cycle have been described to be coordinated with light and temperature to guide swarming in *Anopheles* [80]. Aggregation pheromones have also been described in *A. aegypti* (Fawaz et al., 2014). Interestingly, *Aedes* swarming does not require swarming before mate and *Aedes* mosquitoes have been shown to mate in pairs throughout the day [81].

Upon mating, male sperm is transferred to a spermatheca (one in *Anopheles,* two in *Aedes*) where it is stored for the lifetime of the female mosquito. The role of odorant receptors in activating spermatozoa flagella has been previously shown [82]. While several candidate agonists were shown to activate flagellar beating, its physiological ligand remains to be further defined. Upon insemination, females are thought to mate once in their lifetime. In most *Anopheles* species, this is enforced by the formation of a mating plug that forms a barrier to prevent further female insemination [83]. The mating plug is composed of seminal secretions produced by the male accessory glands [84], and 20-hydroxyecdysone (20E) embedded is thought to play a signaling role in inducing monogamy in the female [26]. While a mating plug is not formed in *Aedes,* a physical barrier is temporarily formed by components of the male sperm produced at the male accessory gland [85]. Later, bioactive proteins collectively known as matrone can modulate female behavior at the neuronal levels and induce monogamy [86, 87]. Nevertheless, the exact molecular composition of matrone remains to be defined. A further understanding of the molecular basis for male-induced monogamy is of great importance, as it could potentially identify chemicals that could be used (e.g., in aerosols) to prevent virgin female mating.

3.6 Sterile insect technique (SIT)

General models from the middle of the twentieth century had already predicted the potential of releasing sterile male releases to suppress insect populations [88]. This approach known as the sterile insect technique (SIT) has been originally accomplished by irradiation of mosquitoes. Sterile animals have been released, mostly by preliminary investigations, in several locations around the world with varied success, as previously discussed [89]. While claims of reduced competitive rates of irradiated mosquitoes are still a matter of debate [90], the biggest issues facing SIT seem to rely on the scalability and sustainability of such efforts [89]. An alternative approach has been the release of transgenic-induced sterile mosquitoes. Still, the logistic challenges of such practices remain a major challenge for field implementations in large geographic areas, with wild-type mosquito populations rapidly returning after release interruption [91]. At present, the development of efficient and flexible gene drive techniques, such as CRISPR/Cas9, remains a promising approach to the development of efficient cost-effective SIT implementations independent of continuous mosquito release [92].

3.7 *Wolbachia*-induced cytoplasmic incompatibility

The utilization of *Wolbachia*-induced cytoplasmic incompatibility remains one of the most promising alternatives for insecticide-independent strategies of vector control. *Wolbachia* is an arthropod-specific bacteria that establish a systemic infection and can be vertically transmitted by infecting the host oocytes [93]. Several strains of *Wolbachia* are known to induce a phenomenon known as cytoplasmic incompatibility (CI) where the progeny from infected males and uninfected females are turned nonviable [94]. While recent reports have identified populations of *A. aegypti* carrying native *Wolbachia* infections [95], these seem to be deviations from a general rule where *Wolbachia* strains are not naturally able to infect *A. aegypti*. Nevertheless, *Wolbachia* strains have previously been adapted to infect *A. aegypti* by trans-infection in the lab, and CI has been shown to manifest in this model. In that sense, the release of CI-carrying *Wolbachia*-infected males has been proposed as a strategy to suppress *Aedes* populations, and field trials have been implemented [96, 97]. The molecular mechanisms mediating cytoplasmic incompatibility started to be elucidated and two key genes linked with the prophage WO have been identified [98, 99]. Transgenesis of such genes would provide alternatives to induce CI in the absence of *Wolbachia* infections [100]. Such strategies would be beneficial for the cases where stable *Wolbachia* trans-infections have not been achieved, as is the case of many anophelines.

4. Concluding remarks

The control of vector populations has shrunk the map of many vector-borne diseases [10, 101], but new strategies will need to be developed to continue this process. Although the fundamental biology behind oocyte development is known and mostly conserved, its molecular mechanisms are still to be explored. The recent completion of multiple genome sequencing projects will allow comparative genomics studies that not only increase our knowledge about reproductive processes but also facilitate the identification of novel species-specific targets for vector control. Research directed to understanding how this process is regulated and being able to manipulate the female's capacity to produce so many viable eggs will lead to safe and effective ways to block reproduction in blood-feeding insects. To accomplish this, there is an urgent need to integrate the post-genomics findings with the species-specific vectors' physiology. Such tactics are the safest path to unravel evidence-based information and design customized tools to manage vector populations in different endemic areas.

Acknowledgements

This work was funded by the following grants. Fundação Carlos Chagas Filho De Amparo À Pesquisa Do Estado Do Rio De Janeiro (FAPERJ) (JCNE E-26/2031802017; http://www.faperj.br/) to I.R.; Conselho Nacional de Desenvolvimento Científico e Tecnológico (CNPq) (INCT-EM 16/2014; http://cnpq.br/) to I.R.; Coordenação de Aperfeiçoamento de Pessoal de Nível Superior (CAPES) (https://www.gov.br/capes/pt-br) to I.R. The authors thank Vinicius Torrão for the excellent technical assistance with the illustration design.

Conflict of interest

The funders had no role in study design, data collection, analysis, and decision to publish, or preparation of the manuscript.

Author details

Isabela Ramos[1]* and Fabio Gomes[2]

1 Instituto de Bioquímica Médica Leopoldo de Meis (IBqM), Universidade Federal do Rio de Janeiro (UFRJ), Rio de Janeiro, Brazil

2 Instituto de Biofísica Carlos Chagas Filho (IBCCF), Universidade Federal do Rio de Janeiro (UFRJ), Rio de Janeiro, Brazil

*Address all correspondence to: isabela@bioqmed.ufrj.br

References

[1] Bhatt S, Gething PW, Brady OJ, Messina JP, Farlow AW, Moyes CL, et al. The global distribution and burden of dengue. Nature. 2013;**496**:504. DOI: 10.1038/nature12060

[2] Pan American Health Organization. Annual epidemiological update for Dengue, Chikungunya and Zika in 2020. 2020. Available from: https://www.paho.org/en

[3] Mlakar J, Korva M, Tul N, Popović M, Poljšak-Prijatelj M, Mraz J, et al. Zika virus associated with microcephaly. The New England Journal of Medicine. 2016;**374**:951-958. DOI: 10.1056/NEJMOA1600651/SUPPL_FILE/NEJMOA1600651_DISCLOSURES.PDF

[4] de Araújo TVB, de Ximenes RA, de Miranda-Filho D, Souza WV, Montarroyos UR, de Melo AP, et al. Association between microcephaly, zika virus infection, and other risk factors in Brazil: Final report of a case-control study. The Lancet Infectious Diseases. 2018;**18**:328-336. DOI: 10.1016/S1473-3099(17)30727-2

[5] Álvarez-Hernández D-A, García-Rodríguez-Arana R, Ortiz-Hernández A, Álvarez-Sánchez M, Wu M, Mejia R, et al. A systematic review of historical and current trends in Chagas disease. Therapeutic Advanced Infectious Diseases. 2021;**8**:20499361211033716. DOI: 10.1177/20499361211033715

[6] Sachs J, Malaney P. The economic and social burden of malaria. Nature. 2002;**415**:680-685

[7] Shepard DS, Coudeville L, Halasa YA, Zambrano B, Dayan GH. Economic impact of dengue illness in the Americas. The American Journal of Tropical Medicine and Hygiene. 2011;**84**:200-207. DOI: 10.4269/AJTMH.2011.10-0503

[8] Caminade C, McIntyre KM, Jones AE. Impact of recent and future climate change on vector-borne diseases. Annals of the New York Academy of Sciences. 2019;**1436**:157-173. DOI: 10.1111/NYAS.13950

[9] Iwamura T, Guzman-Holst A, Murray KA. Accelerating invasion potential of disease vector *Aedes aegypti* under climate change. Nature Communication. 2020;**111**:1-10

[10] Wilson AL, Courtenay O, Kelly-Hope LA, Scott TW, Takken W, Torr SJ, et al. The importance of vector control for the control and elimination of vector-borne diseases. PLoS Neglected Tropical Diseases. 2020;**14**:1-31. DOI: 10.1371/journal.pntd.0007831

[11] Attardo GM, Hansen IA, Raikhel AS. Nutritional regulation of vitellogenesis in mosquitoes: Implications for anautogeny. Insect Biochemistry and Molecular Biology. 2005;**35**:661-675. DOI: 10.1016/j.ibmb.2005.02.013

[12] Shaw WR, Attardo GM, Aksoy S, Catteruccia F. A comparative analysis of reproductive biology of insect vectors of human disease. Current Opinion in Insect Science. 2015;**10**:142-148. DOI: 10.1016/j.cois.2015.05.001

[13] Lange AB, Leyria J, Orchard I. The hormonal and neural control of egg production in the historically important model insect , *Rhodnius prolixus* : A review , with new insights in this post-genomic era. General and Comparative Endocrinology. 2022:322

[14] Rivera-Pérez C, Clifton ME, Noriega FG, Jindra M. Juvenile hormone regulation and action. Advances in invertebrate (neuro) endocrinology. Apple Academic Press; 2020:1-76

[15] Zou Z, Saha TT, Roy S, Shin SW, Backman TWH, Girke T, et al. Juvenile hormone and its receptor, methoprene-tolerant, control the dynamics of mosquito gene expression. Proceedings of the National Academy of Sciences of the United States of America. 2013;**110**:E2173-E2181. DOI: 10.1073/pnas.1305293110

[16] Davey KG. Some consequences of copulation in Rhodnius prolixus. Journal of Insect Physiology. 1967;**13**:1629-1636. DOI: 10.1016/0022-1910(67)90158-8

[17] Davey KG. Effect of the brain and corpus cardiacum on egg production in Rhodnius prolixus. Archives of Insect Biochemistry and Physiology. 1987;**4**:243-249

[18] Davey KG, Maimets I-K, Ruegg RP. The relationship between crop size and egg production in Rhodnius prolixus. Canadian Journal of Zoology. 1986;**64**:2654-2657. DOI: 10.1139/z86-385

[19] Davey KG. Inputs to the hormonal control of egg development in Rhodnius prolixus. Memórias do Instituto Oswaldo Cruz. 1987;**82**:103-108

[20] Borovsky D, Carlson DA, Hancock RG, Rembold H, Van Handel E. De novo biosynthesis of juvenile hormone III and I by the accessory glands of the male mosquito. Insect Biochemistry and Molecular Biology. 1994;**24**:437-444. DOI: 10.1016/0965-1748(94)90038-8

[21] Clifton ME, Correa S, Rivera-Perez C, Nouzova M, Noriega FG. Male Aedes aegypti mosquitoes use JH III transferred during copulation to influence previtellogenic ovary physiology and affect the reproductive output of female mosquitoes. Journal of Insect Physiology. 2014;**64**:40-47. DOI: 10.1016/j.jinsphys.2014.03.006

[22] Klowden MJ. Mating and nutritional state affect the reproduction of Aedes albopictus mosquitoes. Journal of American Mosquito Control Association. 1993;**9**:169-173

[23] Klowden MJ, Chambers GM. Male accessory gland substances activate egg development in nutritionally stressed Aedes aegypti mosquitoes. Journal of Insect Physiology. 1991;**37**:721-726. DOI: 10.1016/0022-1910(91)90105-9

[24] Shaw WR, Teodori E, Mitchell SN, Baldini F, Gabrieli P, Rogers DW, et al. Mating activates the heme peroxidase HPX15 in the sperm storage organ to ensure fertility in Anopheles gambiae. Proceedings of the National Academy of Sciences. USA. 2014;**111**:5854-5859. DOI: 10.1073/pnas.1401715111

[25] Baldini F, Gabrieli P, South A, Valim C, Mancini F, Catteruccia F. The interaction between a sexually transferred steroid hormone and a female protein regulates oogenesis in the malaria mosquito Anopheles gambiae. PLoS Biology. 2013;**11**:e1001695-e1001695. DOI: 10.1371/JOURNAL.PBIO.1001695

[26] Gabrieli P, Kakani EG, Mitchell SN, Mameli E, Want EJ, Mariezcurrena Anton A, et al. Sexual transfer of the steroid hormone 20E induces the postmating switch in Anopheles gambiae. Proceedings of the National Academy of Sciences of the United States of America. 2014;**111**:16353-16358. DOI: 10.1073/pnas.1410488111

[27] Pascual A, Vilardo ES, Taibo C, Sabio García J, Pomar RR. Bicaudal C is

required for the function of the follicular epithelium during oogenesis in Rhodnius prolixus. Development Genes and Evolution. 2021;**231**:33-45. DOI: 10.1007/s00427-021-00673-0

[28] Walter-Nuno AB, Oliveira MP, Oliveira MF, Gonçalves RL, Ramos IB, Koerich LB, et al. Silencing of maternal heme-binding protein causes embryonic mitochondrial dysfunction and impairs embryogenesis in the blood sucking insect rhodnius prolixus. The Journal of Biological Chemistry. 2013;**288**:29323-29332. DOI: 10.1074/jbc.M113.504985

[29] Walter-Nuno AB, Taracena ML, Mesquita RD, Oliveira PL, Paiva-Silva GO. Silencing of iron and heme-related genes revealed a paramount role of iron in the physiology of the hematophagous vector Rhodnius prolixus. Frontiers in Genetics. 2018;**9**:1-21. DOI: 10.3389/fgene.2018.00019

[30] Raikhel AS, Dhadialla TS. Accumulation of yolk proteins in insect oocytes. Annual Review of Entomology. 1992;**37**:217-251. DOI: 10.1146/annurev.en.37.010192.001245

[31] Roy S, Saha TT, Zou Z, Raikhel AS. Regulatory pathways controlling female insect reproduction. Annual Review of Entomology. 2018;**63**:489-511. DOI: 10.1146/annurev-ento-020117-043258

[32] Anderson KL, Woodruff RI. A gap junctionally transmitted epithelial cell signal regulates endocytic yolk uptake in Oncopeltus fasciatus. Developmental Biology. 2001;**239**:68-78. DOI: 10.1006/dbio.2001.0433

[33] Postlethwait JH, Giorgi F. Vitellogenesis in insects. Developmental Biology. 1985;**1985**(1):85-126

[34] Raikhel AS, Dhadialla TS, Cho W-L, Hays AR, Koller CN. Biosynthesis and endocytosis of yolk proteins in the mosquito, in molecular insect science. Hagedorn HH, Hildebrand JG, Kidwell MG, Law JH, editors. Boston, MA: Springer US; 1990:147-154. DOI: 10.1007/978-1-4899-3668-4_18

[35] Brooks RA, Woodruff RI. Calmodulin transmitted through gap junctions stimulates endocytic incorporation of yolk precursors in insect oocytes. Developmental Biology. 2004;**271**:339-349

[36] Ferenz H-J. Receptor-mediated endocytosis of insect yolk proteins. In: Hagedorn HH, Hildebrand JG, Kidwell MG, Law JH, editors. Molecular Insect Science. Boston, MA: Springer US; 1990. pp. 131-138. DOI: 10.1007/978-1-4899-3668-4_16

[37] Richard DS, Gilbert M, Crum B, Hollinshead DM, Schelble S, Scheswohl D. Yolk protein endocytosis by oocytes in Drosophila melanogaster: Immunofluorescent localization of clathrin, adaptin and the yolk protein receptor. Journal of Insect Physiology. 2001;**47**:715-723. DOI: 10.1016/S0022-1910(00)00165-7

[38] Raikhel AS, Dhadialla TS, Cho W-L, Hays AR, Koller CN. Biosynthesis and endocytosis of yolk proteins in the mosquito. In: Hagedorn HH, Hildebrand JG, Kidwell MG, Law JH, editors. Molecular Insect Science. Boston, MA: Springer US; 1990. pp. 147-154. DOI: 10.1007/978-1-4899-3668-4_18

[39] Vieira PH, Benjamim CF, Atella GC, Ramos I. VPS38/UVRAG and ATG14, the variant regulatory subunits of the ATG6/Beclin 1-PI3K complexes, are crucial for the biogenesis of the yolk organelles and are transcriptionally regulated in the oocytes of the vector Rhodnius prolixus. PLoS Neglected Tropical Diseases. 2021;**1**:1

[40] Vieira PH, Bomfim L, Atella GC, Masuda H, Ramos I. Silencing of RpATG6 impaired the yolk accumulation and the biogenesis of the yolk organelles in the insect vector *R. prolixus*. PLoS Neglected Tropical Diseases. 2018;**12**:1-19. DOI: 10.1371/journal.pntd.0006507

[41] Papantonis A, Swevers L, Iatrou K. Chorion genes: A landscape of their evolution, structure, and regulation. Annual Review of Entomology. 2015;**60**:177-194. DOI: 10.1146/annurev-ento-010814-020810

[42] Marinotti O, Ngo T, Kojin BB, Chou SP, Nguyen B, Juhn J, et al. Integrated proteomic and transcriptomic analysis of the Aedes aegypti eggshell. BMC Developmental Biology. 2014;**14**:1-11. DOI: 10.1186/1471-213X-14-15

[43] Han Q, Li G, Li J. Purification and characterization of chorion peroxidase from Aedes aegypti eggs. Archives of Biochemistry and Biophysics. 2000;**378**:107-115. DOI: 10.1006/abbi.2000.1821

[44] Li JS, Li J. Major chorion proteins and their crosslinking during chorion hardening in Aedes aegypti mosquitoes. Insect Biochemistry and Molecular Biology. 2006;**36**:954-964. DOI: 10.1016/j.ibmb.2006.09.006

[45] Fang J, Han Q, Johnson JK, Christensen BM, Li J. Functional expression and characterization of Aedes aegypti dopachrome conversion enzyme. Biochemical and Biophysical Research Communications. 2002;**290**:287-293. DOI: 10.1006/bbrc.2001.6200

[46] Johnson JK, Li J, Christensen BM. Cloning and characterization of a dopachrome conversion enzyme from the yellow fever mosquito, *Aedes aegypti*. Insect Biochemeical and Moecularl Biology. 2001;**31**:1125-1135. DOI: 10.1016/s0965-1748(01)00072-8

[47] Kim SR, Yao R, Han Q, Christensen BM, Li J. Identification and molecular characterization of a prophenoloxidase involved in Aedes aegypti chorion melanization. Insect Molecular Biology. 2005;**14**:185-194. DOI: 10.1111/j.1365-2583.2004.00547.x

[48] Li JS, Li J. Characterization of N-linked oligosaccharides in chorion peroxidase of Aedes aegypti mosquito. Protein Science. 2005;**14**:2370-2386. DOI: 10.1110/ps.051419105

[49] Ferdig MT, Li J, Severson DW, Christensen BM. Mosquito dopa decarboxylase cDNA characterization and blood-meal-induced ovarian expression. Insect Molecular Biology. 1996;**5**:119-126. DOI: 10.1111/j.1365-2583.1996.tb00046.x

[50] Isoe J, Koch LE, Isoe YE, Rascón AA, Brown HE, Massani BB, et al. Identification and characterization of a mosquito-specific eggshell organizing factor in Aedes aegypti mosquitoes. PLoS Biology. 2019;**17**:1-23. DOI: 10.1371/journal.pbio.3000068

[51] Wang Z, Liu P, Inuzuka H, Wei W. Roles of F-box proteins in cancer. Nature Reviews. Cancer. 2014;**14**:233-247. DOI: 10.1038/nrc3700

[52] Dias FA, Gandara AC, Carolin P, Queiroz-Barros FG, RLL O, MHF S, et al. Ovarian dual oxidase (Duox) activity is essential for insect eggshell hardening and waterproofing. The Journal of Biological Chemistry. 2013;**288**:35058-35067. DOI: 10.1074/jbc.M113.522201

[53] Bomfim L, Vieira P, Fonseca A, Ramos I. Eggshell ultrastructure and delivery of pharmacological inhibitors to the early embryo of R . prolixus

by ethanol permeabilization of the extraembryonic layers. PLoS One. 2017;**12**:e0185770. DOI: 10.1371/journal.pone.0185770

[54] Beament JWL. The waterproofing process in eggs of Rhodnius prolixus Stähl. Proceedings of the Royal Society of London. 1946;**133**:407-418

[55] Bouts DMD, Melo AC, Andrade AL, Silva-Neto MA, de Paiva-Silva SMH, et al. Biochemical properties of the major proteins from Rhodnius prolixus eggshell. Insect Biochemistry and Molecular Biology. 2007;**37**:1207-1221. DOI: 10.1016/j.ibmb.2007.07.010

[56] Medeiros MN, Logullo R, Ramos IB, Sorgine MHF, Paiva-Silva GO, Mesquita RD, et al. Transcriptome and gene expression profile of ovarian follicle tissue of the triatomine bug rhodnius prolixus. Insect Biochemistry and Molecular Biology. 2011;**41**:823-831. DOI: 10.1016/j.ibmb.2011.06.004

[57] Bomfim L, Ramos I. Deficiency of ULK1/ATG1 in the follicle cells disturbs ER homeostasis and causes defective chorion deposition in the vector Rhodnius prolixus. FASEB Journal of Official Publication. 2020;**34**:13561-13572. DOI: 10.1096/fj.202001396R

[58] Rios T, Bomfim L, Ramos I. The transition from vitellogenesis to choriogenesis triggers the downregulation of the UPR sensors IRE1 and PERK and alterations in the ER architecture in the follicle cells of the vector Rhodnius prolixus. Cell and Tissue Research. 2022;**387**:63-74. DOI: 10.1007/s00441-021-03547-z

[59] Santos A, Ramos I. ATG3 is important for the chorion ultrastructure during oogenesis in the insect vector Rhodnius prolixus. Frontiers in Physiology. 2021;**12**:1-11. DOI: 10.3389/fphys.2021.638026

[60] Pereira J, Dias R, Ramos I. Knockdown of E1- and E2-ubiquitin enzymes triggers defective chorion biogenesis and modulation of autophagy-related genes in the follicle cells of the vector Rhodnius prolixus. Journal of Cellular Physiology. 2022;**1**:12

[61] Farnesi LC, Menna-Barreto RFS, Martins AJ, Valle D, Rezende GL. Physical features and chitin content of eggs from the mosquito vectors Aedes aegypti, Anopheles aquasalis and Culex quinquefasciatus: Connection with distinct levels of resistance to desiccation. Journal of Insect Physiology. 2015;**83**:43-52. DOI: 10.1016/j.jinsphys.2015.10.006

[62] Rezende GL, Martins AJ, Gentile C, Farnesi LC, Pelajo-Machado M, Peixoto AA, et al. Embryonic desiccation resistance in Aedes aegypti: Presumptive role of the chitinized serosal cuticle. BMC Developmental Biology. 2008;**8**:1-14

[63] Moreira MF, dos Santos AS, Marotta HR, Mansur JF, Ramos IB, Machado EA, et al. A chitin-like component in Aedes aegypti eggshells, eggs and ovaries. Insect Biochemistry and Molecular Biology. 2007;**37**:1249-1261. DOI: 10.1016/j.ibmb.2007.07.017

[64] Mansur JF, Figueira-Mansur J, Santos AS, Santos-Junior H, Ramos IB, de Medeiros MN, et al. The effect of lufenuron, a chitin synthesis inhibitor, on oogenesis of Rhodnius prolixus. Pesticide Biochemistry and Physiology. 2010;**98**:59-67. DOI: 10.1016/j.pestbp.2010.04.013

[65] Souza-Ferreira PS, Mansur JF, Berni M, Moreira MF, Dos Santos RE, Araújo HMM, et al. Chitin deposition on the embryonic cuticle of Rhodnius prolixus: The reduction of CHS transcripts by CHS-ds RNA injection

in females affects chitin deposition and eclosion of the first instar nymph. Insect Biochemistry and Molecular Biology. 2014;**51**:101-109. DOI: 10.1016/j.ibmb.2013.12.004

[66] Mansur JF, Alvarenga ESL, Figueira-Mansur J, Franco TA, Ramos IB, Masuda H, et al. Effects of chitin synthase double-stranded RNA on molting and oogenesis in the Chagas disease vector Rhodnius prolixus. Insect Biochemistry and Molecular Biology. 2014;**51**:110-121. DOI: 10.1016/j.ibmb.2013.12.006

[67] Wigglesworth VB. Source of moulting hormone in Rhodnius. Nature. 1951;**168**:558. DOI: 10.1038/168558b0

[68] Wigglesworth VB. Factors controlling moulting and 'metamorphosis' in an insect. Nature. 1934;**133**:725-726. DOI: 10.1038/133725b0

[69] Buxton PA. The biology of a blood-sucking bug, Rhodnius prolixus. Transaction on Entomological Society of London. 1930;**78**

[70] Wigglesworth VB. The Principles of Insect Physiology. 7th ed. London: Chapman and Hall ltda; 1979. DOI: 10.1007/978.94.009.5973-6

[71] Ahmed AM, Hurd H. Immune stimulation and malaria infection impose reproductive costs in *Anopheles gambiae* via follicular apoptosis. Immun. Infect. 2006;**8**:308-315. DOI: 10.1016/j.micinf.2005.06.026

[72] Medeiros MN, Ramos IB, Oliveira DMP, da Silva RCB, Gomes FM, Medeiros LN, et al. Microscopic and molecular characterization of ovarian follicle atresia in Rhodnius prolixus Stahl under immune challenge. Journal of Insect Physiology. 2011;**57**:945-953. DOI: 10.1016/j.jinsphys.2011.04.010

[73] Samaddar S, Marnin L, Butler LR, Pedra JHF. Immunometabolism in arthropod vectors: Redefining interspecies relationships. Trends in Parasitology. 2020;**36**:807-815. DOI: 10.1016/J.PT.2020.07.010

[74] Mitchell SN, Catteruccia F. Anopheline reproductive biology: Impacts on Vectorial capacity and potential avenues for malaria control. Cold Spring Harbor Perspectives in Medicine. 2017;**7**:a025593-a025593. DOI: 10.1101/CSHPERSPECT.A025593

[75] Atella GC, Bittencourt-Cunha PR, Nunes RD, Shahabuddin M, Silva-Neto MAC. The major insect lipoprotein is a lipid source to mosquito stages of malaria parasite. Acta Tropica. 2009;**109**:159-162. DOI: 10.1016/J.ACTATROPICA.2008.10.004

[76] Werling K, Shaw WR, Itoe MA, Westervelt KA, Marcenac P, Paton DG, et al. Steroid hormone function controls non-competitive plasmodium development in Anopheles. Cell. 2019;**177**:315-325. DOI: 10.1016/J.CELL.2019.02.036

[77] Costa G, Gildenhard M, Eldering M, Lindquist RL, Hauser AE, Sauerwein R, et al. Non-competitive resource exploitation within mosquito shapes within-host malaria infectivity and virulence. NatureCommunication. 2018;**9**:1-11

[78] Rono MK, Whitten MMA, Oulad-Abdelghani M, Levashina EA, Marois E. The major yolk protein vitellogenin interferes with the anti-plasmodium response in the malaria mosquito Anopheles gambiae. PLoS Biology. 2010;**8**:e1000434-e1000434. DOI: 10.1371/JOURNAL.PBIO.1000434

[79] Mozūraitis R, Hajkazemian M, Zawada JW, Szymczak J, Pålsson K,

Sekar V, et al. Male swarming aggregation pheromones increase female attraction and mating success among multiple African malaria vector mosquito species. Nature Ecological and Evolution. 2020;**410**:1401-1395

[80] Wang G, Vega-Rodríguez J, Diabate A, Liu J, Cui C, Nignan C, et al. Clock genes and environmental cues coordinate Anopheles pheromone synthesis, swarming, and mating. Science. 2021;**371**:411-415. DOI: 10.1126/SCIENCE.ABD4359

[81] Hartberg WK. Observations on the mating behaviour of *Aedes aegypti* in nature. Bulletin World Health Organ. 1971;**45**:847

[82] Pitts RJ, Liu C, Zhou X, Malpartida JC, Zwiebel LJ. Odorant receptor-mediated sperm activation in disease vector mosquitoes. Proceedings of the National Academy of Sciences. 2014;**111**:2566-2571. DOI: 10.1073/pnas.1322923111

[83] Mitchell SN, Kakani EG, South A, Howell PI, Waterhouse RM, Catteruccia F. Evolution of sexual traits influencing vectorial capacity in anopheline mosquitoes. Science. 2015;**347**:985-988. DOI: 10.1126/science.1259435

[84] Rogers DW, Baldini F, Battaglia F, Panico M, Dell A, Morris HR, et al. Transglutaminase-mediated semen coagulation controls sperm storage in the malaria mosquito. PLoS Biology. 2009;7:e1000272-e1000272. DOI: 10.1371/JOURNAL.PBIO.1000272

[85] Spielman A Sr, Leahy MG, Skaff V. Seminal loss in repeatedly mated female Aedes aegypti. The Biological Bulletin. 1967;**132**:404-412

[86] Fuchs MS, Craig GB, Hiss EA. The biochemical basis of female monogamy in mosquitoes: I. extraction of the active principle from *Aedes aegypti*. Life Sciences. 1968;7:835-839. DOI: 10.1016/0024-3205(68)90114-8

[87] Gwadz RW. Neuro-hormonal regulation of sexual receptivity in female Aedes aegypti. Journal of Insect Physiology. 1972;**18**:259-266. DOI: 10.1016/0022-1910(72)90126-6

[88] Knipling EF. Possibilities of insect control or eradication through the use of sexually sterile males. Journal of Economic Entomology. 1955;**48**:459-462. DOI: 10.1093/JEE/48.4.459

[89] Benedict MQ. Sterile insect technique: Lessons from the past. Journal of Medical Entomology. 2021;**58**:1974-1979. DOI: 10.1093/JME/TJAB024

[90] Bouyer J, Vreysen MJB. Yes, irradiated sterile male mosquitoes can Be sexually competitive! Trends in Parasitology. 2020;**36**:877-880. DOI: 10.1016/J.PT.2020.09.005

[91] Garziera L, Pedrosa MC, de Souza FA, Gómez M, Moreira MB, Virginio JF, et al. Effect of interruption of over-flooding releases of transgenic mosquitoes over wild population of Aedes aegypti: Two case studies in Brazil. Entomologia Experimentalis et Applicata. 2017;**164**:327-339. DOI: 10.1111/EEA.12618

[92] Macias VM, Ohm JR, Rasgon JL. Gene drive for mosquito control: Where did it come from and where are we headed? International Journal of Environmental Research and Public Health. 2017;**14**:1006

[93] Kaur R, Shropshire JD, Cross KL, Leigh B, Mansueto AJ, Stewart V, et al. Living in the endosymbiotic world of Wolbachia: A centennial review. Cell Host & Microbe. 2021;**29**:879-893. DOI: 10.1016/j.chom.2021.03.006

[94] Sicard M, Bonneau M, Weill M. Wolbachia prevalence, diversity, and ability to induce cytoplasmic incompatibility in mosquitoes. Current Opinion in Insect Science. 2019;**34**:12-20. DOI: 10.1016/J.COIS.2019.02.005

[95] Balaji S, Jayachandran S, Prabagaran SR. Evidence for the natural occurrence of Wolbachia in Aedes aegypti mosquitoes. FEMS Microbiology Letters. 2019;**366**:55. DOI: 10.1093/FEMSLE/FNZ055

[96] Beebe NW, Pagendam D, Trewin BJ, Boomer A, Bradford M, Ford A, et al. Releasing incompatible males drives strong suppression across populations of wild and Wolbachia-carrying Aedes aegypti in Australia. Proceedings of the National Academy of Sciences of the United States of America. 2021;**118**:2106828118. DOI: 10.1073/PNAS.2106828118/SUPPL_FILE/PNAS.2106828118.SAPP.PDF

[97] Crawford JE, Clarke DW, Criswell V, Desnoyer M, Cornel D, Deegan B, et al. Efficient production of male Wolbachia-infected *Aedes aegypti* mosquitoes enables large-scale suppression of wild populations. Nature Biotechnology. 2020;**38**:482

[98] Beckmann JF, Ronau JA, Hochstrasser M. A Wolbachia deubiquitylating enzyme induces cytoplasmic incompatibility. Nature Microbiology. 2017;**25**(2):1-7. DOI: 10.1038/nmicrobiol.2017.7

[99] Le Page DP, Metcalf JA, Bordenstein SR, On J, Perlmutter JI, Shropshire JD, et al. Prophage WO genes recapitulate and enhance Wolbachia-induced cytoplasmic incompatibility. Nature. 2017;**543**:243-274

[100] Adams KL, Abernathy DG, Willett BC, Selland EK, Itoe MA, Catteruccia F. Wolbachia cif B induces cytoplasmic incompatibility in the malaria mosquito vector. Natural Microbiology. 2021;**6**:1575-1582

[101] Shaw WR, Catteruccia F. Vector biology meets disease control: Using basic research to fight vector-borne diseases. Nature Microbiology. 2019;**4**:20-34. DOI: 10.1038/s41564-018-0214-7

Section 2

Eco-epidemiology and Physiopathology

Chapter 3

Neglected Arboviruses in Latin America

Alfonso J. Rodriguez-Morales and D. Katterine Bonilla-Aldana

Abstract

Over the last decade, there has been an increasing concern for epidemics in Latin America, as well as in other regions, due to arboviruses causing epidemics. Before 2013, dengue and yellow fever were of major preoccupation in urban and rural areas, respectively. But after that year, the emergence of chikungunya (2013) and Zika (2015) with their widespread in the region, affected millions of individuals, especially in tropical countries. Nowadays, other alpha and flaviviruses, but also bunyaviruses, have been circulating in the region causing small outbreaks, as is the case of Mayaro, Madariaga, Rocio, Oropouche, and St. Louis encephalitis, among others. In the current chapter, we address the situation regarding these other arboviruses that have been neglected by also being a differential diagnosis and an etiology of febrile syndrome in the region.

Keywords: Mayaro, Madariaga, Rocio, Oropouche, St. Louis encephalitis, alphavirus, flavivirus, neglected, Latin America

1. Introduction

Vector-borne diseases and many zoonotic diseases remain significantly relevant in tropical areas, such as Latin America. In the specific case of those caused by viruses, arboviruses, this region, as well as Asia, are particularly affected over time, primarily due to the widespread of competent vectors, as is the case of *Aedes aegypti*, but also *A. albopictus*, and more recently *A. vittatus* [1, 2]. Then, as expected, an integrated One Health approach, considering the environment, and animal and human health, is needed for vector-borne diseases [3].

Over the last decades, multiple arboviral diseases caused by alphaviruses and flaviviruses have been a concern in Latin America [4]. However, since the introduction of yellow fever and dengue, the epidemiological landscape in the region has significantly changed [5]. Dutch slave traders brought yellow fever (YFV) to the America from Africa during the mid-seventeenth century.

For the next two and a half centuries, the disease terrorized seaports throughout the America [6]. Reports describe the possible first introduction in 1648 in Mexico [5, 7–9]. Although some studies suggest dengue (DENV) was introduced in the America, through the Caribbean islands in 1635 [5, 10, 11], before 1981, dengue was considered a public health problem only in Asia and posed little or no threat to the region of the America [11, 12]. This scenario shifted with the 1981 Cuban epidemic, the first significant dengue epidemic in the area. For the following decade, sporadic cases of dengue were observed. Then, in 1990, Venezuela experienced the second major epidemic in the region. These events marked dengue as an emerging disease in the America [11, 12]. As observed, flaviviruses, such as dengue and yellow fever, have been significant concerns regarding morbidity and mortality in the region [4, 13–27]. Additionally, many of them, as observed with Zika (ZIKV) and chikungunya (CHIKV), lead to chronic consequences, such as central nervous system (CNS) compromise (including congenital microcephaly and other complications of congenital Zika syndrome) [28–32], as well as chronic rheumatic and non-rheumatic diseases (CHIKV) [33–39].

Taxonomically speaking, the essential arboviruses are included in the genus alphavirus, family Togaviridae (**Figure 1**), which consists of a total of 32 species; and in the genus flavivirus, family Flaviviridae (**Figure 2**), where 53 species are currently included.

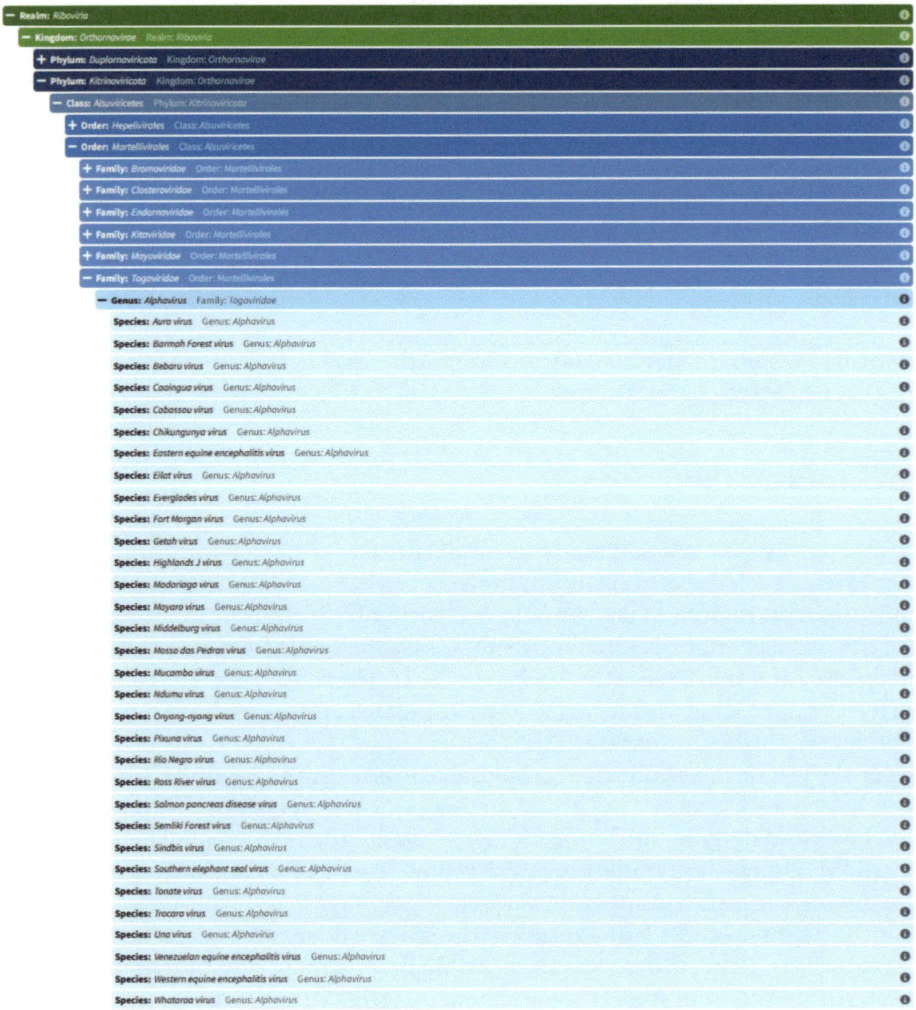

Figure 1.
Taxonomical classification of viruses belonging to the genus alphavirus (family Togaviridae, order martellivirales, class alsuviricetes). (https://ictv.global/taxonomy).

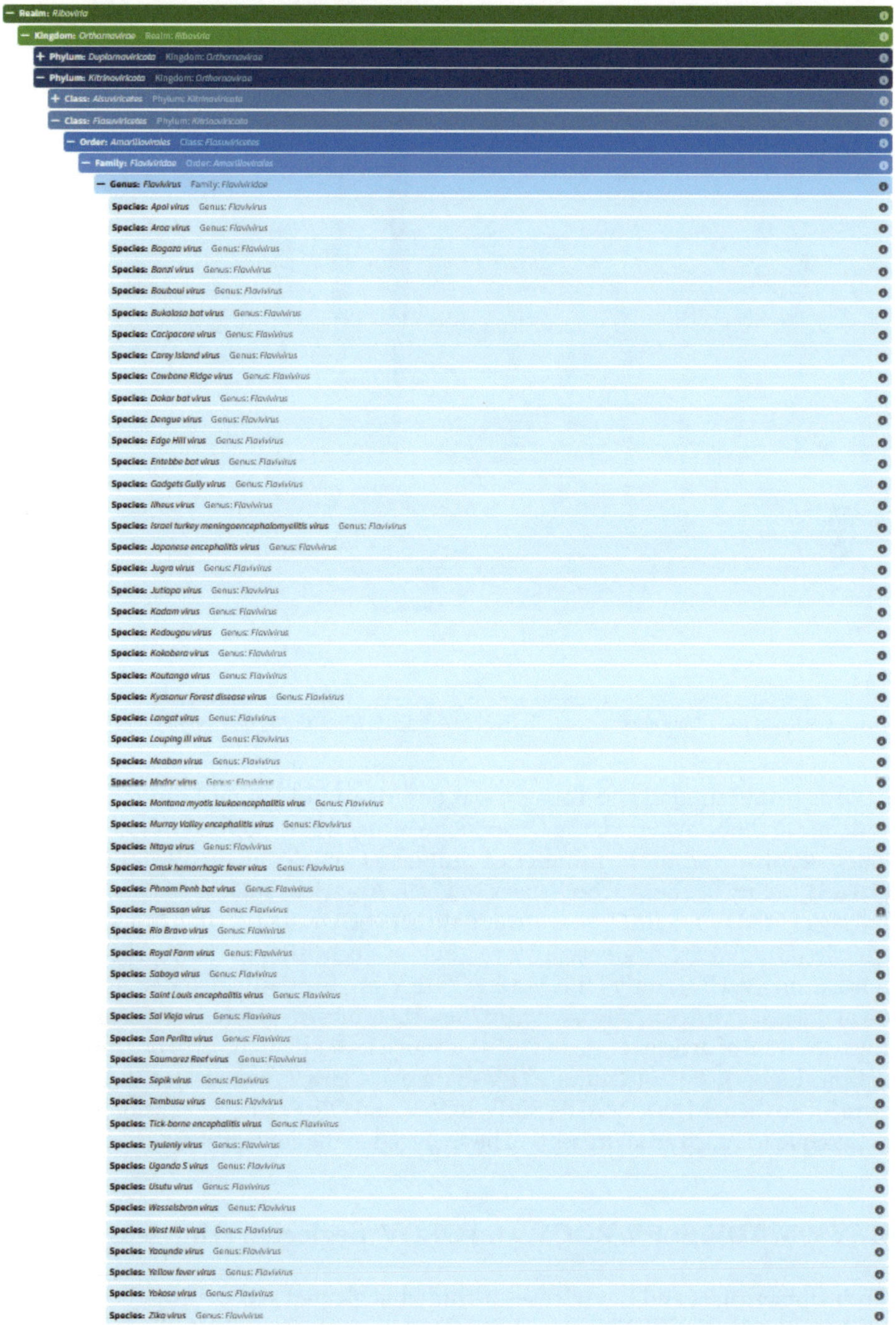

Figure 2.
Taxonomical classification of viruses belonging to the genus flavivirus (family Flaviviridae, order amarillovirales, class flasuviricetes). (https://ictv.global/taxonomy).

Alphaviruses, originally endemic in Latin America, such as the Venezuelan equine encephalitis (VEE) and the eastern equine encephalitis; were described in 1920 in Venezuela and 1972 in Trinidad and Tobago, respectively [5]. Mayaro virus, another

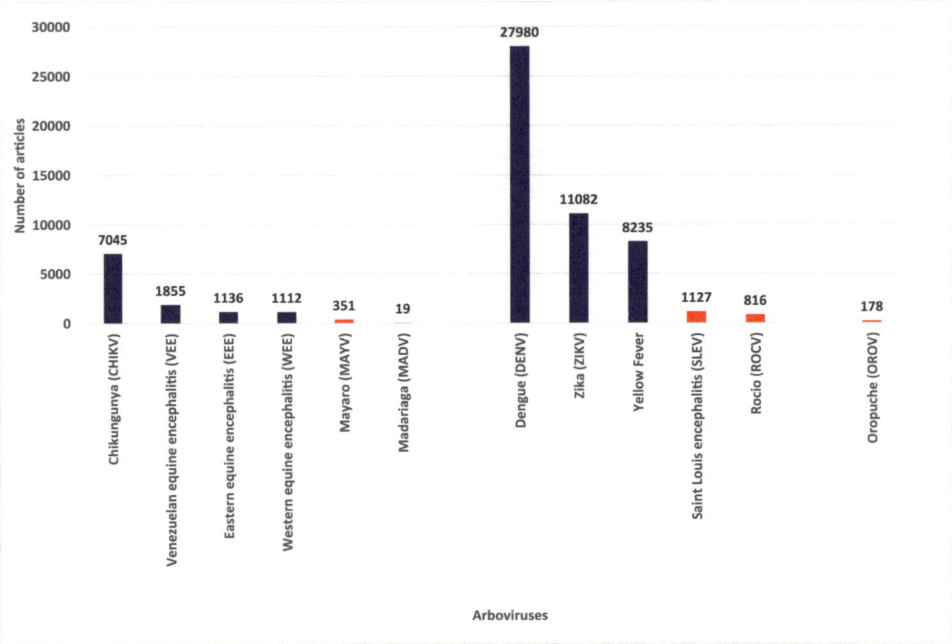

Figure 3.
The number of articles published about arboviruses (alphaviruses, flaviviruses, and orthobunyaviruses) in Latin America, cumulated until November 1, 2022, in PubMed-indexed journals. (https://pubmed.ncbi.nlm.nih.gov/).

alphavirus from Trinidad and Tobago, was described in 1954. In Trinidad and Tobago, an endemic orthobunyavirus, the Oropouche virus, was described in 1955 [5].

Then, as observed in the number of published articles available in PubMed (**Figure 3**), many of these arboviruses in Latin America, such as Mayaro (MAYV), Madariaga (MADV), Saint Louis encephalitis (SLEV), Rocio (ROCV), and Oropuche (OROV) are neglected. Nevertheless, according to the World Health Organization (WHO), only DENV and CHIKV are formally included as neglected tropical diseases (https://www.who.int/health-topics/neglected-tropical-diseases).

Even the total of articles of them (1364) is much lower than the total of DENV (20.5 times higher), ZIKV (8 times), YFV (6 times), CHIKV (5 times), or VEE (1.4 times) (**Figure 3**). So then, MAYV, MADV, SLEV, ROCV, and OROV may be considered neglected. As a consequence, such arboviruses will be analyzed in the current chapter.

2. MAYV, MADV, SLEV, ROCV, and OROV: neglected arboviruses

Both alphaviruses and flaviviruses included neglected arboviruses. Nevertheless, given the importance of DENV and YFV, flaviviruses have been studied more, and even vaccines for a long time have existed for YFV [25] and recently for DENV [40]. However, there are no vaccines against alphaviruses for humans. Nevertheless, after epidemics of CHIKV in 2014–2015 in the America, their importance increased. However, as a group, the situation is worse regarding investigating orthobunyaviruses. Epidemics of CHIKV and ZIKV, as well as periodical outbreaks of YFV, especially in Brazil and Venezuela, have influenced the attention and research on these alphaviruses and flaviviruses [26, 27].

The region's MAYV, MADV, SLEV, ROCV, and OROV can be considered neglected arboviruses [41–44]. Even in most countries, such arboviruses are not under regular surveillance, laboratory investigation, and confirmation.

2.1 Mayaro (MAYV)

MAYV, an enzootic virus [44, 45], is an alphavirus that shares epidemiological features with YFV, having sylvatic cycles involving animal reservoirs and with sylvatic and urban mosquito vectors. Clinically, MAYV shares characteristics with its genus and family. It is an arthritogenic alphavirus, as occurs with CHIKV, able to generate immune-mediated chronic disease [46, 47] but overlaps in symptoms during the acute phase with other arboviruses [48]. A few years ago, the ChikDenMaZika syndrome was proposed as a mnemotechnic rule to keep in mind Mayaro and other more frequently observed arboviruses, such as CHIKV, DENV, and ZIKV [48]. That would help decrease the negligence of Mayaro, to be considered in the differential diagnosis of febrile syndrome in the tropics or possibly caused by an arbovirus. MAYV is more frequently detected in other countries, in addition to Trinidad and Tobago, Brazil, and Peru. It has also been identified in Panama, French Guiana, Colombia, Argentina, Venezuela, and Paraguay [49, 50]. Studies have reported MAYV positivity in wild mammals, birds, or reptiles, as well as in domestic animals. Also, 12 orders of wild-caught vertebrates, most frequently in Charadriiformes and primate orders, have been identified with MAYV. This alphavirus has been detected in wild-caught mosquito genera, including *Haemagogus*, *Aedes*, *Culex*, *Psorophora*, *Coquillettidia*, and *Sabethes* [49]. Although MAYV has been identified in urban vectors, there is no evidence of sustained urban transmission. MAYV's enzootic cycle could become established in forested areas within cities, similar to the yellow fever virus [51]. Arboviruses in mosquito body pools sampled during the rainy season of 2018 in 21 bird-watching points of Cuiabá and Varzea Grande, south central Mato Grosso, Brazil, highlights the possibility of MAYV detection in urban areas of Latin America [52]. An investigation of arboviruses in patients with acute febrile illness (n=453) for less than 5 days in Mato Grosso state during the period of ZIKV and CHIKV dissemination in Brazil found multiple other neglected arboviruses [53]. Alphaviruses were detected in 2 (0.4%) patients infected with CHIKV genotype ECSA, 1 (0.2%) with Madariaga (EEEV) lineage III, and 34 (7.5%) with Mayaro (MAYV) genotype L. Four (11.4%) patients presented dual infections with DENV-1/ZIKV, DENV-1/DENV4, DENV-4/MAYV, and ZIKV/MAYV. The majority—13/34 positive for MAYV, one for Madariaga virus—are residents in Várzea Grande, the metropolitan region of Cuiabá, the capital of Mato Grosso [53]. Up to June 2015, only 121 articles were published in PubMed-indexed journals, based on a bibliometric analysis [47]. After 7 years, only 230 additional papers have been published on MAYV (**Figure 3**).

In countries, such as Peru, MAYV has become more critical in epidemiological terms; even MAYV is under surveillance in that country (**Figure 4**). Although that, there is still a lack of research from that country in MAYV (only 28 articles, <8% of the total on MAYV in PubMed). Especially in jungle areas in the country's north and south border with Brazil, Peru has endemic areas where MAYV and other arboviruses cause infection.

During 2017–2020, a total of 36 cases were reported by Peru (**Table 1**), most of them (29, 81%) in 2017 and predominantly in the Madre de Dios department (16, 44%) that year (**Table 1**). At least seven departments of Peru, from a total of 24, reported at least one case of MAYV during that period.

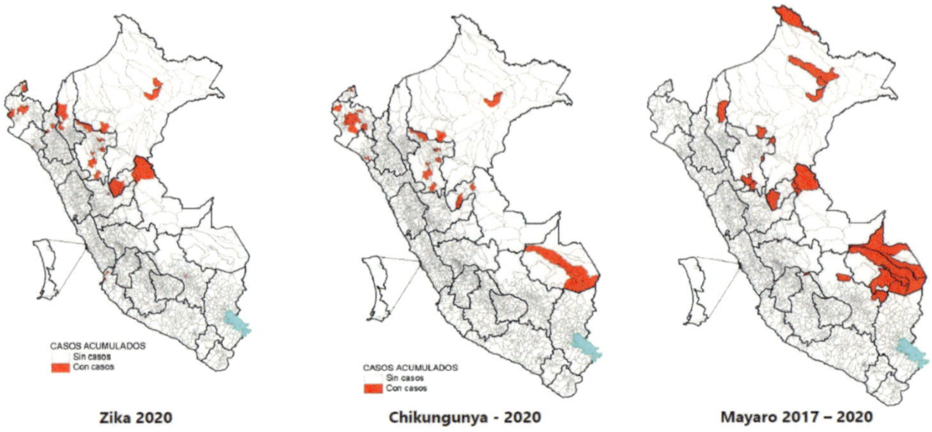

Figure 4.
Geographical distribution of ZIKV, CHIKV, and MAYV in Peru, 2020. (Modified from https://www.dge.gob.pe/epipublic/uploads/boletin/boletin_202043.pdf).

2.2 Oropouche (OROV)

In Peru, there is limited detection of OROV, an orthobunyavirus. But in 2016, at least in three districts of Madre de Dios (2) and Cusco (1), OROV outbreaks were detected (Tambopata, Iñapari, and Ocobamba).

OROV is another neglected arbovirus [54]. OROV is a species in the genus orthobunyavirus, the family Peribunyaviridae (**Figure 5**). That genus includes 103 species, but only OROV is considered of medical importance in Latin America. More relevant in North America, this genus contains the La Cross virus (LACV), which has not yet been identified in Latin America [55].

In another bibliometric study performed in June 2015 [54], only 83 articles were recovered from PubMed (43% from Brazil, 18% from the United States of America, and 6% from Peru) [54]. On May 2016, the Ministry of Health of Peru reported 57 cases of OROV [54]. Cases of OROV have also been reported in nearby countries, such as Panama, Ecuador, French Guiana, Haiti, Suriname, Trinidad and Tobago, Brazil, and Venezuela [56–60]. As occurs with MAYV, OROV is under surveillance in Peru but not in most countries of Latin America. After 7 years of the unique bibliometric assessment of OROV so far [54], only 95 additional articles have been published, showing clearly the lack of research on this orthobunyavirus.

Nevertheless, recent studies (2021–2022) in Colombia have identified OROV as an emerging cause of acute febrile illness in the country [61]. In a study with 2,967 individuals, OROV was identified in 87 of 791 (10.9%) viremic cases, where an RT-qPCR dual-target assay was possible. Those cases were from Cali (the third largest city in the country) (3/53), Cucuta (border with Venezuela) (3/19), Villavicencio (easter lowlands) (38/566), and Leticia (Amazon jungle) (43/153). In parallel, an automated anti-nucleocapsid antibody assay detected IgM in 27/503 (5.4%) and IgG in 92/568 (16.2%) patients screened, for which 24/68 (35.3%) of PCR positives had antibodies [61]. Such findings confirm OROV as an emerging pathogen and recommend increased surveillance to determine its burden as a cause of acute febrile illness in Colombia [61]. A previous assessment in Colombia diagnosed OROV in a woman 28 years of age from Turbaco, Bolivar department (near Cartagena), by viral isolation, quantitative reverse transcription PCR, and phylogenetic analysis of the small,

	Cases per year				%				Incidence (cases/100,000 pop.)			
Departments	**2017**	**2018**	**2019**	**2020**	**2017**	**2018**	**2019**	**2020**	**2017**	**2018**	**2019**	**2020**
Madre de Dios	16	0	0	0	55.17	0	0	0	11.14	0	0	0
Loreto	3	0	3	1	10.34	0	50	100	0.28	0	0.28	0.1
San Martin	5	0	0	0	17.24	0	0	0	0.06	0	0	0
Ucayali	4	0	0	0	13.79	0	0	0	0.08	0	0	0
Cusco	0	0	2	0	0	0	33.33	0	0	0	0.15	0
Amazonas	1	0	0	0	3.45	0	0	0	0.24	0	0	0
Ayacucho	0	0	1	0	0	0	16.67	0	0	0	0.14	0
Total	29	0	6	1	100	0	100	100	0.09	0	0.02	0.003

(Modified from https://www.dge.gob.pe/epipublic/uploads/boletin/boletin_202043.pdf).

Table 1.
Cases of MAYV in Peru, 2017–2020.

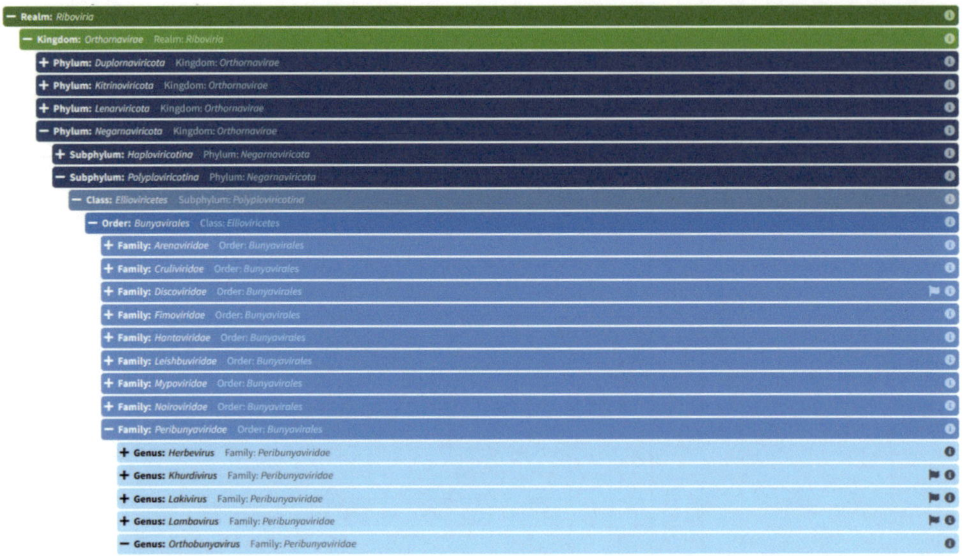

Figure 5.
Taxonomical location of the genus orthobunyavirus (family Peribunyaviridae). (https://ictv.global/taxonomy).

medium, and large genomic segments. That virus was related to a strain isolated in Ecuador in 2016 [62]. That means that in countries, such as Colombia, OROV should be considered in the differential diagnosis of fever and investigated as part of the surveillance [45, 63], especially in possibly endemic areas.

2.3 Saint Louis encephalitis virus (SLEV)

Saint Louis encephalitis virus (SLEV) is a flavivirus, a member of the Japanese encephalitis virus serogroup, initially identified in 1933 in Saint Louis, Missouri, USA, as encephalitis lethargica [64], during an outbreak involving 475 cases with 71 deaths (14.9%) [65]. The encephalitis lethargica occurred in Saint Louis in 1919, 1924, and 1932 [65]. Studies on SLEV in Latin America also lack, regardless of its epidemiological situation [66]. In a bibliometric study performed in December 2016 [64], only 955 articles were recovered from PubMed (44% from the United States of America, 4% from Brazil, and 4% from Argentina) [64]. After 6 years of that bibliometric assessment of SLEV, only 172 additional articles have been published, clearly showing the lack of research on this flavivirus.

Culex species generally transmit SLEV as vectors and birds as animal hosts. Most SLEV infections are asymptomatic, but clinical manifestations range from nonspecific febrile syndrome to febrile headache, aseptic meningitis, and encephalitis, with fatality ranging from 3 to 30% [67]. In the case of Latin America, SLEV is one of the flaviviruses that circulate in Brazil [68]. Reports from Argentina [69, 70], Colombia [71], Cuba [72], Ecuador [73], French Guiana [74], Guatemala [75], Mexico [76], Panama [67, 77], Peru [78], and Uruguay [79] have also been published, among other possible identifications in other Latin countries. The primary SLEV mosquito vectors in some endemic areas include *Culex tarsalis*, *C. pipiens*, and *C. quinquefasciatus* [80, 81]. Like most arboviruses that cause central nervous system (CNS) disease in humans, most SLEV infections are asymptomatic or mild, with symptom onset 5–15 days after exposure and exhibiting a broad range of clinical presentations [80].

	Arboviruses				
Clinical findings	**MAYV**	**MADV**	**ROCV**	**OROV**	**SLEV**
Fever/chills	++++	+	++	++	+++
Myalgia/arthralgia/fatigue	+++	++	0	++	+/0
Edema in limbs	0	0	0	0	0
Maculopapular rash	++	0	0	0	0
Retro-ocular pain	++	0	0	0	+/0
Conjunctivitis, non-purulent	0	0	+	0	0
Lymphadenopathies	+	0	0	0	0
Hepatomegaly	+	0	0	0	0
Leukopenia/thrombocytopenia	++	0	0	0	0
Encephalitis	0	++	++	0	++++
Meningitis	0	0/+	++	0	+++
Headache	0	++	++	++	+++
Photophobia	0	0	0	+++	++
Hemorrhages	0	0	0	0	0

MAYV, Mayaro; MADV, Madariaga; ROCV, Rocio; OROV, Oropouche; SLEV, St. Louis Encephalitis.

Table 2.
Clinical findings of neglected arboviruses in Latin America and the proposed mnemotechnic of **MAMA-ROS** *syndrome (***MA***yaro,* **MA***dariaga,* **R***ocio,* **O***ropouche and* **S***t. Louis encephalitis).*

The discussed neglected arboviruses may overlap clinically, then, initial differentiation between them, may be complex (**Table 2**). Unfortunately, major infectious and tropical diseases books do not cover some of them (e.g., MADV) [82, 83].

2.4 Madariaga (MADV)

Recent ecologic and genetic studies of eastern equine encephalitis virus (EEEV; togaviridae: alphavirus) have demonstrated clear separation between North and South American EEEV strains: North American EEEV cluster in a single genetic lineage—lineage I, in the system proposed by Arrigo et al. [84]—with South American EEEV strains (now known as Madariaga virus [MADV]) clustering in EEEV lineages II, III, and IV. Although there is a reasonable understanding of North American EEE's clinical and epidemiologic features, much less is known about MADV infections. MADV is neglected in multiple ways [85]. Contrasting with other neglected arboviruses, MADV has no previous bibliometric assessments nor for EEE. As shown before, there is a significant lack of studies about it [85–94]. Recent studies in Panama have clinically characterized this emerging encephalitis (**Table 2**) [90]. Studies from that central American countries suggest that the lack of additional neurological cases may indicate that severe MADV infections occur only rarely. Field studies suggest that over the past five decades, alphavirus infections, such as MADV and VEEV, have occurred at low levels in eastern Panama, but that MADV and VEEV infections have recently increased-potentially during the past decade. In some of eastern Panama, the endemic diseases and outbreaks of MADV and VEEV appear to differ spatially [95].

These neglected arboviruses are usually neglected; in the past, the ChikDenMaZika syndrome helped to decrease the neglect of thinking on Mayaro. Nevertheless, still, that alphavirus, as well as others, and the rest of discussed arboviruses, should be considered for an additional mnemotechnic, as **MAMA-ROS** syndrome (**MA**yaro, **MA**dariaga, **R**ocio, **O**ropouche and **S**t. Louis encephalitis) (**Table 2**) to think in them as differential diagnoses, as also to assess their clinical presentations.

2.5 Rocio (ROCV)

ROCV emerged as a cause of outbreaks of encephalitis in Brazil during 1975–1976. However, as another neglected arbovirus, there are less than 1,000 articles in PubMed (**Figure 3**), with no bibliometric studies.

After initial descriptions, sporadic reports have been identified; nevertheless, no additional outbreaks have been reported. ROCV is probably circulating among wild birds and transmitted by *Psorophora ferox* and *Aedes scapularis* [82, 83]. It has an incubation period of 7–14 days, and illness begins with headache, fever, nausea, and vomiting, sometimes with pharyngitis and conjunctivitis (**Table 2**). Meningitis or encephalitis follows in many, with altered mental state and cerebellar tremor. Convulsions are uncommon. The case fatality rate is about 10%. Death occurs in patients of all ages with neurological sequelae. Gait disturbances may appear in survivors [1, 2]. Some of these neglected viruses are commonly detected during dengue outbreaks, as with other arboviruses. Patients result negative for DENV and are investigated for multiple other flaviviruses and alphaviruses. Recent seroprevalence studies in animals detected ROCV in regions of Brazil, indicating risk for reemergence of this pathogen. A recent study identified ROCV RNA in samples from two human patients for whom dengue fever was clinically suspected but ruled out by laboratory findings. Then, such results suggest that testing for infrequent flavivirus infections should be considered, including ROCV [96, 97].

A group of maps showing the distribution by countries where neglected arboviruses have been reported (**Figure 6**). Theses maps do not necessarily reflect the real distribution, but just countries that have published cases or studies showing arboviral circulation. In the case of countries, such as Bolivia and Paraguay, is particularly curious that they have not reported most of the neglected arboviral pathogens, although have been described in most of their neighboring countries.

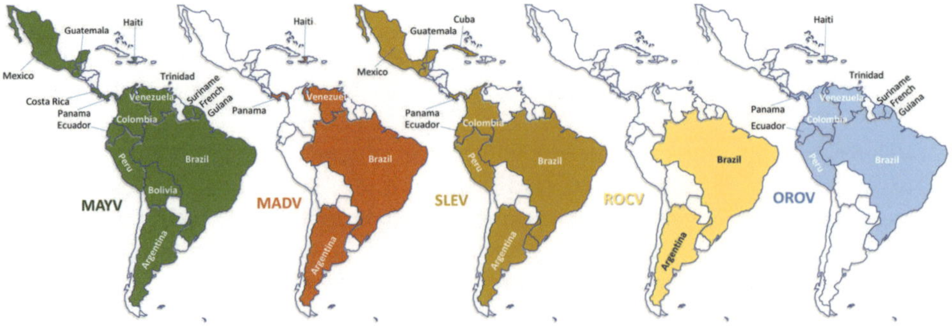

Figure 6.
Distribution map of MAYV, MADV, ROCV, OROV, and SLEV in Latin America. This distribution indicates just circulation in the country, but not necessarily that has been detected nationwide.

		Vector						
		Aedes	***Culex***	***Culicoides***	***Haemagogus***	***Psorophora***	***Coquillettidia***	***Sabethes***
Arbovirus	MAYV	x	x		x	x	x	x
	MADV	?	x			x		
	ROCV	x	?			x		
	OROV	x	x	x				
	SLEV	?	x					

x, studies have reported the detection of the arbovirus; ?, potential vector.

Table 3.
Main reported vectors of neglected arboviruses in Latin America.

A significant problem in the diagnosis of these arboviruses includes the clinical and epidemiological overlapping [4], even with possible coinfections [16, 22, 98], but also the problems derived from potential antibody cross-reactivity that may yield serological false-positive results, now even, including coinfections and cross-reactivity with SARS-CoV-2 [18, 99–102]. Then, molecular diagnosis of them is critical, including multiplex testing to search simultaneously many arboviruses and perform more specific serological testing, using better antigens, such as plaque reduction neutralizing antibody testing (PRNT) [103], especially in patients with risks for severe or complicated disease.

For the control of these neglected arboviruses, vector control is key, especially on *Aedes* and *Culex* species that represent the main mosquito genuses related to their transmission (**Table 3**).

As expected, no vaccines nor antivirals have been developed for these neglected arboviruses [104–106], although there is hope for them in the future. Therefore, symptomatic treatment is indicated with them after establishing a specific and confirmed molecular diagnosis.

3. Conclusions

Vector-borne diseases, particularly those involving virus transmission, continue to be a significant public health problem, especially in tropical countries, but even with climate change in also in subtropical countries. Still, in multiple countries, problems related to accurate diagnosis of the etiology of febrile syndrome are complex. That is in large magnitude related to arboviral pathogens, many of them neglected, as the case of MAYV, MADV, ROCV, OROV, and SLEV, among others. Therefore, after considering major arboviral diseases, such as DENV, CHIKV, ZIKV, YFV, VEE, and EEE, among others, epidemiological and clinical suspicion of them is critical to establishing a differential diagnosis, detecting them, and even identifying possible coinfections. At the same time, as there is a significant gap in knowledge about neglected arboviruses in Latin America, more research is needed to understand their implications and acute and non-acute clinical consequences and impacts.

Conflicts of interest

AJRM has been a consultant/advisor for Takeda, Sanofi Pasteur, Merck Sharp and Dohme, Valneva, and AstraZeneca.

Author details

Alfonso J. Rodriguez-Morales[1,2,3,4*] and D. Katterine Bonilla-Aldana[5]

1 Grupo de Investigación Biomedicina, Faculty of Medicine, Fundación Universitaria Autónoma de las Américas, Pereira, Risaralda, Colombia

2 Universidad Cientifica del Sur, Lima, Peru

3 Gilbert and Rose-Marie Chagoury School of Medicine, Lebanese American University, Beirut, Lebanon

4 Universidad Privada Franz Tamayo (UNIFRANZ), Cochabamba, Bolivia

5 Research Unit, Universidad Continental, Huancayo, Peru

*Address all correspondence to: alfonso.rodriguez@uam.edu.co

References

[1] Pagac BB, Spring AR, Stawicki JR, Dinh TL, Lura T, Kavanaugh MD, et al. Incursion and establishment of the Old World arbovirus vector Aedes (Fredwardsius) vittatus (Bigot, 1861) in the Americas. Acta Tropica. 2021;**213**:105739

[2] Rodriguez-Morales AJ, Paniz-Mondolfi AE, Faccini-Martínez ÁA, Henao-Martínez AF, Ruiz-Saenz J, Martinez-Gutierrez M, et al. The constant threat of zoonotic and vector-borne emerging tropical diseases: Living on the edge. Frontiers in Tropical Diseases. 2021;**2**:676905

[3] Faburay B. The case for a 'one health' approach to combating vector-borne diseases. Infectious Ecology Epidemiology. 2015;**5**:28132

[4] Rodriguez-Morales AJ, Villamil-Gomez WE, Franco-Paredes C. The arboviral burden of disease caused by co-circulation and co-infection of dengue, chikungunya and Zika in the Americas. Travel Medicine and Infectious Disease. 2016;**14**:177-179

[5] Musso D, Rodriguez-Morales AJ, Levi JE, Cao-Lormeau VM, Gubler DJ. Unexpected outbreaks of arbovirus infections: Lessons learned from the Pacific and tropical America. The Lancet Infectious Diseases. 2018;**18**:e355-ee61

[6] Bryan CS, Moss SW, Kahn RJ. Yellow fever in the Americas. Infectious Disease Clinics of North America. 2004;**18**:275-292

[7] Figueiredo LT. Emergent arboviruses in Brazil. Revista da Sociedade Brasileira de Medicina Tropical. 2007;**40**:224-229

[8] Ortiz-Martinez Y, Patino-Barbosa AM, Rodriguez-Morales AJ. Yellow fever in the Americas: The growing concern about new epidemics. F1000Res. 2017;**6**:398

[9] Rossetto EV, Angerami RN, Luna EJA. What to expect from the 2017 yellow fever outbreak in Brazil? Revista do Instituto de Medicina Tropical de São Paulo. 2017;**59**:e17

[10] Gubler DJ. The changing epidemiology of yellow fever and dengue, 1900 to 2003: Full circle? Comparative Immunology, Microbiology and Infectious Diseases. 2004;**27**:319-330

[11] Brathwaite Dick O, San Martín JL, Montoya RH, del Diego J, Zambrano B, Dayan GH. The history of dengue outbreaks in the Americas. The American journal of tropical medicine and hygiene. 2012;**87**:584-593

[12] Dengue in Central America. The epidemics of 2000. Epidemiological Bulletin. 2000;**21**:4-8

[13] Mattar S, Morales V, Cassab A, Rodriguez-Morales AJ. Effect of climate variables on dengue incidence in a tropical Caribbean municipality of Colombia, Cerete, 2003-2008. International Journal of Infectious Diseases. 2013;**17**:e358-e359

[14] Rodriguez-Morales AJ, Paniz-Mondolfi AE. Venezuela: Far from the path to dengue and chikungunya control. Journal of Clinical Virology. 2015;**66**:60-61

[15] Quintero-Herrera LL, Ramirez-Jaramillo V, Bernal-Gutierrez S, Cardenas-Giraldo EV, Guerrero-Matituy EA, Molina-Delgado AH, et al. Potential impact of climatic variability on the epidemiology of dengue in Risaralda, Colombia, 2010-2011.

Journal of Infection and Public Health. 2015;**8**:291-297

[16] Villamil-Gomez WE, Gonzalez-Camargo O, Rodriguez-Ayubi J, Zapata-Serpa D, Rodriguez-Morales AJ. Dengue, chikungunya and Zika co-infection in a patient from Colombia. Journal of Infection and Public Health. 2016;**9**:684-686

[17] Zambrano LI, Sierra M, Lara B, Rodriguez-Nunez I, Medina MT, Lozada-Riascos CO, et al. Estimating and mapping the incidence of dengue and chikungunya in Honduras during 2015 using Geographic Information Systems (GIS). Journal of Infection and Public Health. 2017;**10**:446-456

[18] Cardona-Ospina JA, Arteaga-Livias K, Villamil-Gomez WE, Perez-DiazCE,KatterineBonilla-AldanaD, Mondragon-Cardona A, et al. Dengue and COVID-19, overlapping epidemics? An analysis from Colombia. Journal of Medical Virology. 2021;**93**(1):522-527. DOI: 10.1002/jmv.26194.

[19] Zambrano LI, Rodriguez E, Espinoza-Salvado IA, Rodriguez-Morales AJ. Dengue in Honduras and the Americas: The epidemics are back! Travel Medicine and Infectious Disease. 2019;**31**:101456

[20] Herrera-Martinez AD, Rodriguez-Morales AJ. Potential influence of climate variability on dengue incidence registered in a western pediatric Hospital of Venezuela. Tropical Biomedicine. 2010;**27**:280-286

[21] Zambrano LI, Sevilla C, Reyes-Garcia SZ, Sierra M, Kafati R, Rodriguez-Morales AJ, et al. Potential impacts of climate variability on dengue hemorrhagic fever in Honduras, 2010. Tropical Biomedicine. 2012;**29**:499-507

[22] Cardona-Ospina JA, Jiménez-Canizales CE, Vásquez-Serna H, Garzón-Ramírez JA, Alarcón-Robayo JF, Cerón-Pineda JA, et al. Fatal dengue, Chikungunya and Leptospirosis: The importance of assessing co-infections in febrile patients in tropical areas. Tropical Medicine and Infectious Disease. 2018;**2018**:3

[23] Rifakis PM, Benitez JA, De-la-Paz-Pineda J, Rodriguez-Morales AJ. Epizootics of yellow fever in Venezuela (2004-2005): An emerging zoonotic disease. Annals of the New York Academy of Sciences. 2006;**1081**:57-60

[24] Rodriguez-Morales AJ, Villamil-Gómez WE. Yellow fever: Still of concern for travelers of Colombia? Infection. 2018;**22**:171-172

[25] Reno E, Quan NG, Franco-Paredes C, Chastain DB, Chauhan L, Rodriguez-Morales AJ, et al. Prevention of yellow fever in travellers: An update. The Lancet Infectious Diseases. 2020;**20**:e129-ee37

[26] Chaves T, Orduna T, Lepetic A, Macchi A, Verbanaz S, Risquez A, et al. Yellow fever in Brazil: Epidemiological aspects and implications for travelers. Travel Medicine and Infectious Disease. 2018;**23**:1-3

[27] Rodríguez-Morales AJ, Bonilla-Aldana DK, Suárez JA, Franco-Paredes C, Forero-Peña DA, Mattar S, et al. Yellow fever reemergence in Venezuela – Implications for international travelers and Latin American countries during the COVID-19 pandemic. Travel Medicine and Infectious Disease. 2021;**2021**:102192

[28] Cardona-Ospina JA, Zapata MF, Grajales M, Arias MA, Grajales J, Bedoya-Rendón HD, et al. Physical growth and neurodevelopment of a cohort of children after 3.5 years of follow-up from mothers with Zika

infection during pregnancy-third report of the ZIKERNCOL Study. Journal of Tropical Pediatrics. 2021;**2021**:67

[29] Villamil-Gomez WE, Guijarro E, Castellanos J, Rodriguez-Morales AJ. Congenital Zika syndrome with prolonged detection of Zika virus RNA. Journal of Clinical Virology. 2017;**95**:52-54

[30] Alvarado-Socarras JL, Idrovo AJ, Contreras-Garcia GA, Rodriguez-Morales AJ, Audcent TA, Mogollon-Mendoza AC, et al. Congenital microcephaly: A diagnostic challenge during Zika epidemics. Travel Medicine and Infectious Disease. 2018;**23**:14-20

[31] Rodriguez-Morales AJ. Zika and microcephaly in Latin America: An emerging threat for pregnant travelers? Travel Medicine and Infectious Disease. 2016;**14**:5-6

[32] Rodriguez-Morales AJ, Cardona-Ospina JA, Ramirez-Jaramillo V, Gaviria JA, Gonzalez-Moreno GM, Castrillon-Spitia JD, et al. Diagnosis and outcomes of pregnant women with Zika virus infection in two municipalities of Risaralda, Colombia: Second report of the ZIKERNCOL study. Travel Medicine and Infectious Disease. 2018;**25**:20-25

[33] Rodriguez-Morales AJ, Cardona-Ospina JA, et al. Prevalence of post-chikungunya infection chronic inflammatory arthritis: A systematic review and meta-analysis. Arthritis Care & Research (Hoboken). 2016;**68**:1849-1858

[34] Rodriguez-Morales AJ, Villamil-Gomez W, Merlano-Espinosa M, Simone-Kleber L. Post-chikungunya chronic arthralgia: A first retrospective follow-up study of 39 cases in Colombia. Clinical Rheumatology. 2016;**35**:831-832

[35] Rodriguez-Morales AJ, Gil-Restrepo AF, Ramirez-Jaramillo V, Montoya-Arias CP, Acevedo-Mendoza WF, Bedoya-Arias JE, et al. Post-chikungunya chronic inflammatory rheumatism: Results from a retrospective follow-up study of 283 adult and child cases in La Virginia, Risaralda, Colombia. F1000Res. 2016;**5**:360

[36] Rodriguez-Morales AJ, Simon F. Chronic chikungunya, still to be fully understood. International Journal of Infectious Diseases. 2019;**86**:133-134

[37] Rodriguez-Morales AJ. Letter to the Editor: Chikungunya virus infection-an update on chronic rheumatism in Latin America. Rambam Maimonides Med Journal. 2017;**2017**:8

[38] Rodriguez-Morales AJ, Restrepo-Posada VM, Acevedo-Escalante N, Rodriguez-Munoz ED, Valencia-Marin M, Castrillon-Spitia JD, et al. Impaired quality of life after chikungunya virus infection: A 12-month follow-up study of its chronic inflammatory rheumatism in La Virginia, Risaralda, Colombia. Rheumatology International. 2017;**37**:1757-1758

[39] Rodriguez-Morales AJ, Calvache-Benavides CE, Giraldo-Gomez J, Hurtado-Hurtado N, Yepes-Echeverri MC, Garcia-Loaiza CJ, et al. Post-chikungunya chronic arthralgia: Results from a retrospective follow-up study of 131 cases in Tolima, Colombia. Travel Medicine and Infectious Diseases. 2016;**14**:58-59

[40] Biswal S, Borja-Tabora C, Martinez Vargas L, Velásquez H, Theresa Alera M, Sierra V, et al. Efficacy of a tetravalent dengue vaccine in healthy children aged 4-16 years: A randomised, placebo-controlled, phase 3 trial. Lancet. 2020;**395**:1423-1433

[41] Pezzi L, Diallo M, Rosa-Freitas MG, Vega-Rua A, Ng LFP, Boyer S, et al. GloPID-R report on chikungunya,

o'nyong-nyong and Mayaro virus, part 5: Entomological aspects. Antiviral Research. 2020;**174**:104670

[42] Pezzi L, LaBeaud AD, Reusken CB, Drexler JF, Vasilakis N, Diallo M, et al. GloPID-R report on chikungunya, o'nyong-nyong and Mayaro virus, part 2: Epidemiological distribution of o'nyong-nyong virus. Antiviral Research. 2019;**172**:104611

[43] Pezzi L, Reusken CB, Weaver SC, Drexler JF, Busch M, LaBeaud AD, et al. GloPID-R report on Chikungunya, O'nyong-nyong and Mayaro virus, part I: Biological diagnostics. Antiviral Research. 2019;**166**:66-81

[44] Pezzi L, Rodriguez-Morales AJ, Reusken CB, Ribeiro GS, LaBeaud AD, Lourenco-de-Oliveira R, et al. GloPID-R report on chikungunya, o'nyong-nyong and Mayaro virus, part 3: Epidemiological distribution of Mayaro virus. Antiviral Research. 2019;**172**:104610

[45] Rodriguez-Morales AJ, Paniz-Mondolfi AE, Villamil-Gomez WE, Navarro JC. Mayaro, Oropouche and Venezuelan Equine Encephalitis viruses: Following in the footsteps of Zika? Travel Medicine and Infectious Disease. 2017;**15**:72-73

[46] Arenivar C, Rodriguez Y, Rodriguez-Morales AJ, Anaya JM. Osteoarticular manifestations of Mayaro virus infection. Current Opinion in Rheumatology. 2019;**31**:512-516

[47] Patino-Barbosa AM, Bedoya-Arias JE, Cardona-Ospina JA, Rodriguez-Morales AJ. Bibliometric assessment of the scientific production of literature regarding Mayaro. Journal of Infection and Public Health. 2016;**9**:532-534

[48] Paniz-Mondolfi AE, Rodriguez-Morales AJ, Blohm G, Marquez M, Villamil-Gomez WE. ChikDenMaZika Syndrome: The challenge of diagnosing arboviral infections in the midst of concurrent epidemics. Annals of Clinical Microbiology and Antimicrobials. 2016;**15**:42

[49] Celone M, Okech B, Han BA, Forshey BM, Anyamba A, Dunford J, et al. A systematic review and meta-analysis of the potential non-human animal reservoirs and arthropod vectors of the Mayaro virus. PLoS Neglected Tropical Diseases. 2021;**15**:e0010016

[50] Mutricy R, Matheus S, Mosnier É, Martinez-Lorenzi E, De Laval F, Nacher M, et al. Mayaro virus infection in French Guiana, a cross sectional study 2003-2019. Infection, Genetics and Evolution. 2022;**99**:105243

[51] Caicedo EY, Charniga K, Rueda A, Dorigatti I, Mendez Y, Hamlet A, et al. The epidemiology of Mayaro virus in the Americas: A systematic review and key parameter estimates for outbreak modelling. PLoS Neglected Tropical Diseases. 2021;**15**:e0009418

[52] da Silva Neves NA, da Silva FR, Morais DO, Pavon JAR, de Pinho JB, Slhessarenko RD. Chikungunya, Zika, Mayaro, and Equine Encephalitis virus detection in adult Culicinae from South Central Mato Grosso, Brazil, during the rainy season of 2018. Brazilian Journal of Microbiology. 2022;**53**:63-70

[53] de Souza Costa MC, Siqueira Maia LM, Costa de Souza V, Gonzaga AM, Correa de Azevedo V, Ramos Martins L, et al. Arbovirus investigation in patients from Mato Grosso during Zika and Chikungunya virus introdution in Brazil, 2015-2016. Acta Tropica. 2019;**190**:395-402

[54] Culquichicón C, Cardona-Ospina JA, Patiño-Barbosa AM,

Rodriguez-Morales AJ. Bibliometric analysis of Oropouche research: Impact on the surveillance of emerging arboviruses in Latin America. F1000Res. 2017;**6**:194

[55] Rogers MB, Gulino KM, Tesh RB, Cui L, Fitch A, Unnasch TR, et al. Characterization of five unclassified orthobunyaviruses (Bunyaviridae) from Africa and the Americas. The Journal of General Virology. 2017;**98**:2258-2266

[56] Navarro JC, Giambalvo D, Hernandez R, Auguste AJ, Tesh RB, Weaver SC, et al. Isolation of Madre de Dios Virus (Orthobunyavirus; Bunyaviridae), an Oropouche Virus Species Reassortant, from a Monkey in Venezuela. The American Journal of Tropical Medicine and Hygiene. 2016;**95**:328-338

[57] Wise EL, Márquez S, Mellors J, Paz V, Atkinson B, Gutierrez B, et al. Oropouche virus cases identified in Ecuador using an optimised qRT-PCR informed by metagenomic sequencing. PLoS Neglected Tropical Diseases. 2020;**14**:e0007897

[58] Elbadry MA, Durães-Carvalho R, Blohm GM, Stephenson CJ, Loeb JC, White SK, et al. Orthobunyaviruses in the Caribbean: Melao and Oropouche virus infections in school children in Haiti in 2014. PLoS Neglected Tropical Diseases. 2021;**15**:e0009494

[59] van Tongeren HA. Occurrence of arboviruses belonging to the C-, Bunyamwera and Guama groups, and of Oropouche, Junin, Tacaiuma and Kwatta viruses in man in the province of Brokopondo, Surinam: A serological survey. Tropical and Geographical Medicine. 1967;**19**:309-325

[60] Gaillet M, Pichard C, Restrepo J, Lavergne A, Perez L, Enfissi A, et al. Outbreak of Oropouche Virus in French Guiana. Emerging Infectious Diseases. 2021;**27**:2711-2714

[61] Ciuoderis KA, Berg MG, Perez LJ, Hadji A, Perez-Restrepo LS, Aristizabal LC, et al. Oropouche virus as an emerging cause of acute febrile illness in Colombia. Emerging Microbes and Infection. 2022;**2022**:1-49

[62] Gómez-Camargo DE, Egurrola-Pedraza JA, Cruz CD, Popuche D, Ochoa-Díaz MM, Guevara C, et al. Evidence of Oropouche Orthobunyavirus Infection, Colombia, 2017. Emerging Infectious Diseases. 2021;**27**:1756-1758

[63] Watts DM, Lavera V, Callahan J, Rossi C, Oberste MS, Roehrig JT, et al. Venezuelan equine encephalitis and Oropouche virus infections among Peruvian army troops in the Amazon region of Peru. The American Journal of Tropical Medicine and Hygiene. 1997;**56**:661-667

[64] Ortiz-Martínez Y, Vega-Useche L, Villamil-Gómez WE, Rodriguez-Morales AJ. Saint Louis Encephalitis Virus, another re-emerging arbovirus: A literature review of worldwide research. Le Infezioni in Medicina. 2017;**25**:77-79

[65] Encephalitis In St. Louis. American Journal of Public Health and the Nation's Health. 1933;**23**:1058-1060

[66] Mansilla AP, Grande JM, Diaz A. Effect of agroecosystems on seroprevalence of St. Louis Encephalitis and West Nile Viruses in Birds, La Pampa, Argentina, 2017-2019. Emerging Infectious Diseases. 2022;**28**:1393-1402

[67] Kopp A, Gillespie TR, Hobelsberger D, Estrada A, Harper JM, Miller RA, et al. Provenance and geographic spread of St. Louis

encephalitis virus. mBio. 2013;**4**: e00322-e00313

[68] Figueiredo LT. The Brazilian flaviviruses. Microbes and infection. 2000;**2**:1643-1649

[69] Batallán GP, Konigheim BS, Quaglia AI, Rivarola ME, Beranek MD, Tauro LB, et al. Autochthonous circulation of Saint Louis encephalitis and West Nile viruses in the Province of La Rioja, Argentina. Review in Argentina Microbiology. 2021;**53**:154-161

[70] Valinotto LE, Barrero PR, Viegas M, Alvarez López MC, Mistchenko AS. Molecular evidence of St. Louis encephalitis virus infection in patients in Buenos Aires, Argentina. Journal of Clinical Virology. 2012;**54**:349-351

[71] Hoyos-López R, Soto SU, Rúa-Uribe G, Gallego-Gómez JC. Molecular identification of Saint Louis encephalitis virus genotype IV in Colombia. Memórias do Instituto Oswaldo Cruz. 2015;**110**:719-725

[72] Pelegrino JL, Suárez M, Guzmán MG, Vázquez S, Benítez NR. Surveillance of St. Louis encephalitis, Eastern equine and Western equine in the province of Ciego de Avila. Revista Cubana de Medicina Tropical. 1996;**48**:109-113

[73] Baquerizo Amador L, Marmol Cevallos F. Serological investigation of St. Louis encephalitis in various regions of Ecuador. Revista Ecuatoriana de Higiene y Medicina Tropical. 1959;**16**:249-259

[74] de Thoisy B, Dussart P, Kazanji M. Wild terrestrial rainforest mammals as potential reservoirs for flaviviruses (yellow fever, dengue 2 and St Louis encephalitis viruses) in French Guiana. Transactions of the Royal Society of Tropical Medicine and Hygiene. 2004;**98**:409-412

[75] Scherer WF, Dickerman RW, Ordóñez JV. Serologic surveys for antibodies to Western, Eastern, California, and St. Louis Encephalitis and Dengue 3 arboviruses in Middle America, 1961-1975. Bulletin of the Pan American Health Organization. 1977;**11**:212-223

[76] Laredo-Tiscareño SV, Garza-HernandezJA, Rodríguez-AlarcónCA, Adame-Gallegos JR, Beristain-Ruiz DM, Barajas-López IN, et al. Detection of antibodies to Lokern, Main Drain, St. Louis Encephalitis, and West Nile Viruses in Vertebrate Animals in Chihuahua, Guerrero, and Michoacán, Mexico. Vector Borne and Zoonotic Diseases. 2021;**21**:884-891

[77] Hayes CG, Dutary BE, Reeves WC, Adames AJ, Galindo P. Experimental studies to determine the susceptibility to infection with St. Louis encephalitis virus of five species of Panamanian mosquitoes. Journal of the American Mosquito Control Association. 1991;**7**:584-587

[78] Felices V, Ampuero JS, Guevara C, Caceda ER, Gomez J, Santiago-Maldonado FW, et al. St. Louis encephalitis virus infection in woman, Peru. Emerging Infectious Diseases. 2014;**20**:730-732

[79] Burgueño A, Spinsanti L, Díaz LA, Rivarola ME, Arbiza J, Contigiani M, et al. Seroprevalence of St. Louis encephalitis virus and West Nile virus (Flavivirus, Flaviviridae) in horses, Uruguay. BioMed Research International. 2013;**2013**:582957

[80] Danforth ME, Snyder RE, Feiszli T, Bullick T, Messenger S, Hanson C, et al. Epidemiologic and environmental characterization of the Re-emergence of St. Louis Encephalitis Virus in California, 2015-2020. PLoS Neglected Tropical Diseases. 2022;**16**:e0010664

[81] Reisen WK. Epidemiology of St. Louis encephalitis virus. Adverse in Virus Research. 2003;**61**:139-183

[82] Markoff L. 153 - Alphaviruses. In: Bennett JE, Dolin R, Blaser MJ, editors. Mandell, Douglas, and Bennett's Principles and Practice of Infectious Diseases. Eighth ed. Philadelphia: W.B. Saunders; 2015. pp. 1865-74.e2

[83] Young PR, Ng LFP, Hall RA, Smith DW, Johansen CA. 14 - Arbovirus Infections. In: Farrar J, Hotez PJ, Junghanss T, Kang G, Lalloo D, White NJ, editors. Manson's Tropical Infectious Diseases. Twenty-third ed. London: W.B. Saunders; 2014. pp. 129-61.e3

[84] Arrigo NC, Adams AP, Weaver SC. Evolutionary patterns of eastern equine encephalitis virus in North versus South America suggest ecological differences and taxonomic revision. Journal of Virology. 2010;**84**:1014-1025

[85] Blohm GM, Lednicky JA, White SK, Mavian CN, Márquez MC, González-García KP, et al. Madariaga virus: Identification of a Lineage III strain in a venezuelan child with acute undifferentiated febrile illness, in the setting of a possible equine epizootic. Clinical Infectious Diseases. 2018;**67**:619-621

[86] Luciani K, Abadia I, Martinez-Torres AO, Cisneros J, Guerra I, Garcia M, et al. Madariaga virus infection associated with a case of acute disseminated encephalomyelitis. The American Journal of Tropical Medicine and Hygiene. 2015;**92**:1130-1132

[87] Stechina OS, Oria GI, Torres C, Diaz LA, Contigiani M, Stein M. First detection of Madariaga virus in Mosquitoes Collected in a Wild Environment of Northeastern Argentina. The American Journal of Tropical Medicine and Hygiene. 2019;**101**:916-918

[88] Buscaglia C. A survey for avian influenza from gulls on the coasts of the District of Pinamar and the Lagoon Salada Grande, General Madariaga, Argentina. Avian Diseases. 2012;**56**:1017-1020

[89] Benvenuto D, Cella E, Fogolari M, De Florio L, Borsetti A, Donati D, et al. The transmission dynamic of Madariaga Virus by bayesian phylogenetic analysis: Molecular surveillance of an emergent pathogen. Microbial Pathogenesis. 2019;**132**:80-86

[90] Carrera JP, Pitti Y, Molares-Martinez JC, Casal E, Pereyra-Elias R, Saenz L, et al. Clinical and serological findings of Madariaga and Venezuelan Equine encephalitis viral infections: A Follow-up Study 5 Years After an Outbreak in Panama. Open Forum Infectious Diseases. 2020;**7**:ofaa359

[91] Gil L, Magalhaes T, Santos B, Oliveira LV, Oliveira-Filho EF, Cunha JLR, et al. Active Circulation of Madariaga Virus, a Member of the Eastern Equine Encephalitis Virus Complex, in Northeast Brazil. Pathogens. 2021;**10**

[92] Lednicky JA, White SK, Mavian CN, El Badry MA, Telisma T, Salemi M, et al. Emergence of Madariaga virus as a cause of acute febrile illness in children, Haiti, 2015-2016. PLoS Neglected Tropical Diseases. 2019;**13**:e0006972

[93] Vittor AY, Armien B, Gonzalez P, Carrera JP, Dominguez C, Valderrama A, et al. Epidemiology of emergent Madariaga Encephalitis in a Region with Endemic Venezuelan Equine Encephalitis: Initial Host Studies and Human Cross-Sectional Study in Darien, Panama. PLoS Neglected Tropical Diseases. 2016;**10**:e0004554

[94] Silva M, Auguste AJ, Terzian ACB, Vedovello D, Riet-Correa F, Macario VMK,

et al. Isolation and characterization of Madariaga virus from a Horse in Paraiba State, Brazil. Transbound Emerging Diseases. 2017;**64**:990-993

[95] Carrera JP, Cucunubá ZM, Neira K, Lambert B, Pittí Y, Liscano J, et al. Endemic and epidemic human alphavirus infections in Eastern Panama: An analysis of population-based cross-sectional surveys. The American Journal of Tropical Medicine and Hygiene. 2020;**103**:2429-2437

[96] Saivish MV, da Costa VG, Rodrigues RL, Féres VCR, Montoya-Diaz E, Moreli ML. Detection of Rocio Virus SPH 34675 during Dengue Epidemics, Brazil, 2011-2013. Emerging Infectious Diseases. 2020;**26**:797-799

[97] Saivish MV, Gomes da Costa V, de Lima MG, Alves da Silva R, Dutra da Silva GC, Moreli ML, et al. Rocio virus: An updated view on an elusive flavivirus. Viruses. 2021;**2021**:13

[98] Villamil-Gómez WE, Rodríguez-Morales AJ, Uribe-García AM, González-Arismendy E, Castellanos JE, Calvo EP, et al. Zika, dengue, and chikungunya co-infection in a pregnant woman from Colombia. International Journal of Infectious Diseases. 2016;**51**:135-138

[99] León-Figueroa DA, Abanto-Urbano S, Olarte-Durand M, Nuñez-Lupaca JN, Barboza JJ, Bonilla-Aldana DK, et al. COVID-19 and dengue coinfection in Latin America: A systematic review. New Microbes New Infections. 2022:101041

[100] Patwary MM, Haque MZ, Bardhan M, Rodriguez-Morales AJ. COVID-19 and Dengue Co-epidemic During the Second Wave of the Pandemic in Bangladesh: A Double Blow for an Overburdened Health-Care System. Disaster Medicine and Public Health Preparedness. 2022;**1-3**

[101] Mejia Buritica L, Karduss Urueta AJ. Pulmonary mucormycosis. The New England Journal of Medicine. 2021;**384**:e69

[102] Villamil-Gómez WE, Rojas-Torres I, Perea-Vásquez LE, Collazos-Torres LA, Murillo-Moreno MA, Morales-Rudas JD, et al. SARS-CoV-2 and Dengue virus co-infection: A case from North Caribbean Colombia. Travel Medicine and Infectious Disease. 2021;**102096**

[103] Cardona-Ospina JA, Trujillo AM, Jiménez-Posada EV, Sepúlveda-Arias JC, Tabares-Villa FA, Altieri-Rivera JS, et al. Susceptibility to endemic Aedes-borne viruses among pregnant women in Risaralda, Colombia. International Journal of Infectious Diseases. 2022;**122**:832-840

[104] da Silva MK, Azevedo AAC, Campos DMO, de Souto JT, Fulco UL, Oliveira JIN. Computational vaccinology guided design of multi-epitope subunit vaccine against a neglected arbovirus of the Americas. Journal of Biomolecular Structure & Dynamics. 2022:1-18

[105] Powers JM, Haese NN, Denton M, Ando T, Kreklywich C, Bonin K, et al. Non-replicating adenovirus based Mayaro virus vaccine elicits protective immune responses and cross protects against other alphaviruses. PLoS Neglected Tropical Diseases. 2021;**15**:e0009308

[106] Darwish MA, Hammon WM. Preparation of inactivated St. Louis encephalitis virus vaccine from hamster kidney cell culture. Proceedings of the Society for Experimental Biology and Medicine Society for Experimental Biology and Medicine (New York, NY). 1966;**123**:242-246

Chapter 4

Mycobacterium ulcerans Disease and Host Immune Responses

Michael S. Avumegah

Abstract

Mycobacterium ulcerans is the causative agent of the subcutaneous necrotic condition known as Buruli ulcer (BU).BU is Neglected Tropical Disease. The bacillus is the third most common mycobacteria disease-causing agent after *Mycobacterium tuberculosis* and *Mycobacterium leprae*. *M. ulcerans* produces the toxin-Mycolactone, which plays a key role in the pathophysiological features of the disease. Buruli ulcer has been reported in 34 countries, mainly in the tropics and subtropics. Tropical countries include Benin, Cameroon, Ghana, Democratic Republic of Congo and Nigeria. BU is also prevalent in Queensland, a subtropical region, and in Victoria, a temperate area, all within Australia. The exact mode of the transmission remains unclear. However, *M. ulcerans* is believed to have an aquatic niche. Initial diagnosis of BU is based on the experience of the clinician, but PCR targeting the *M. ulcerans* DNA, IS2404, isolation and culture of the bacillus and histopathology are used for confirmation. The current, commonly used methods for confirmatory diagnosis have logistic and resource challenges. Novel cell mediated immunity (CMI) and serology-based tests would be beneficial to provide a more accurate assessment of population exposure.

Keywords: *Mycobacterium ulcerans*, Buruli ulcer disease

1. Introduction

Mycobacterium ulcerans is the causative agent of the subcutaneous necrotic condition known as Buruli ulcer (**Figure 1**) [2, 3]. The bacillus is the third most common mycobacteria disease causing agent after *Mycobacterium tuberculosis* and *Mycobacterium leprae* [4].

M. ulcerans produces the toxin-Mycolactone (**Figure 2**), which plays a key role in the pathophysiological features of the disease [6–8]. Buruli ulcer has been reported in 34 countries (**Figure 3**), mainly in the tropics and subtropics [10]. Tropical countries include Benin [11], Cameroon [12–14], Ghana [15], Democratic Republic of Congo [16] and Nigeria [17, 18]. BU is also prevalent in Queensland [19], a subtropical region, and in Victoria, a temperate area, all within Australia [20].

The exact mode of the transmission remains unclear [10, 21]. However, *M. ulcerans* is believed to have an aquatic niche [22–26]. Aquatic insects, belonging to the Family: Belostomatidae and Naucoridae have been implicated as possible vectors in Africa [22, 27, 28]. In Australia, mosquitoes [20] and possum [29] have been suggested as vector and reservoir [20, 29] respectively. Initial diagnosis of BU is based on the

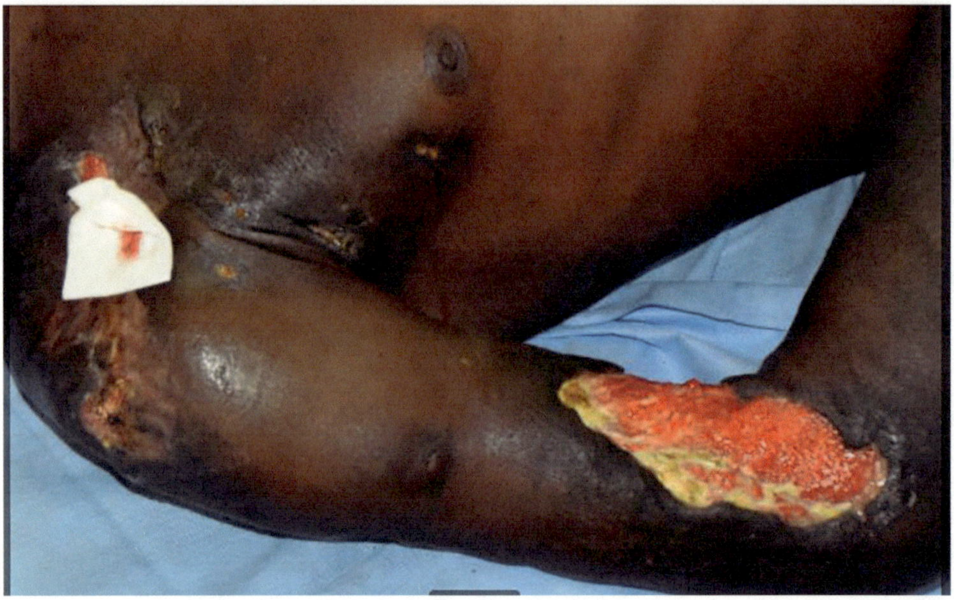

Figure 1.
A severe Buruli ulcer on the upper limb. Image was taken from WHO website [1].

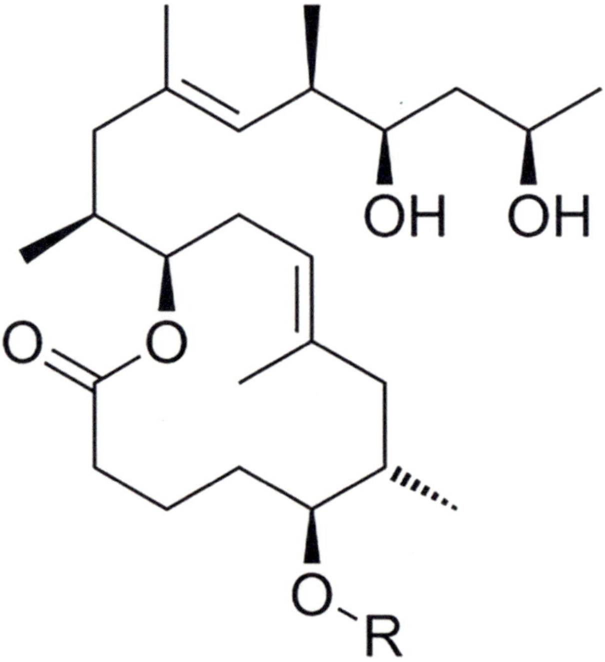

Figure 2.
Mycolactone structure [5].

experience of the clinician [30], but PCR targeting the *M. ulcerans* DNA, IS*2404* [31], isolation and culture of the bacillus and histopathology are used for confirmation [32–34].

DOI: http://dx.doi.org/10.5772/intechopen.103843

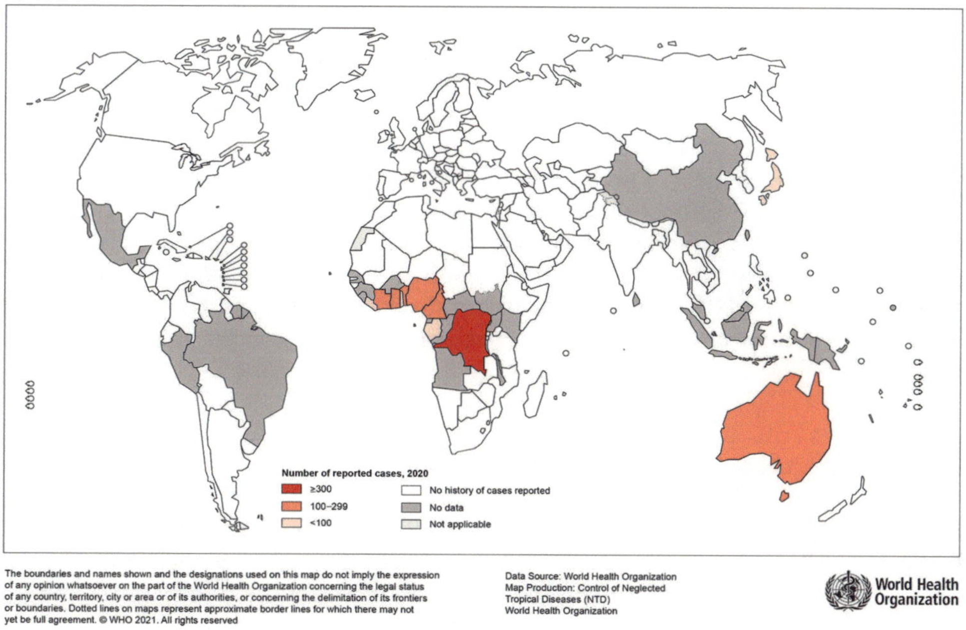

Figure 3.
Distribution of Buruli ulcer, worldwide, 2020 [9].

In Africa, the disease is common in the rural setting where access to medical facilities and other infrastructure is limited [35, 36]. The opposite is true in Australia [10]. More cases have been reported among people living near wetlands [21, 37]. Gender is not a risk factor [10, 38], however age has been identified as a non-environmental risk factor [10, 38]. BU is prevalence among children between 5 and 15 age group in Africa [38]. Whereas in Australia the >60 age group are most susceptible [39–41]. This has been attributed to the ageing population in Australia, as well as immunosenescence [41–43].

2. *Mycobacterium ulcerans* infection

The time of infection or exposure to *M. ulcerans* to showing clinical symptoms of BU ranges from 1 week to 9 months [44]. The median incubation period is 4.5 months [44]. Non-ulcerative and ulcerative are the two main forms of the disease. The non-ulcerative form manifests as either painless nodule, swelling, plaque or oedema [45].

Opened necrotic lesion on the skin describes the ulcerative form and is categorised into 3 forms. Category 1 ulcers are single lesion on the skin and 5 cm in diameter [46]. Ulcers with size 5 to 15 cm is characterised as category 2 [46]. Multiples ulcers on different part of the body and/or ulcers greater than 15 cm is clinically described as category 3 [46]. African cohort usually report category 3 and 2 ulcers whereas category 1 are common in Australia [46]. This has been attributed to differences in geographical strains and virulence factor of *M. ulcerans* [47]. Access to adequate medical services in rural endemic regions in Africa and late presentation of condition to medical centres is another reason [30, 48].

Rook *et al.*, described 3 phases of immune response to *M. ulcerans* in murine model in 1975 [49]. The first phase involves leucocyte migration and delayed hypersensitivity response at the site of infection [49]. This response is usually cell-mediated and involves proliferation of T-cells, monocytes and macrophages. In the next phase, as *M. ulcerans* cells multiple at the site of infection, there is subsequent reduction in the migration of inflammatory biomarkers at this site [49]. Though, there appears to be reactive cells in the lymph nodes [49]. The last phase is marked by depletion of T-cells [49]. This is attributed to excessive exposure to the bacillus toxins (mycolactone) [49]. Studies in tuberculosis and BU patients also confirms that individuals could have a negative skin-test while their lymph tissues is filled with enormous responsive cells [50, 51]. These 3 phases describes the phenomena of "sensitization" and "desensitisation" in mycobacteria infection. The latter being the non-appearances of cell-mediated response to a previously encountered antigen [49, 52].

3. Role of mycolactone in disease progression

Mycolactone is responsible for the necrotic nature of the disease [6, 7]. It is essentially a lipid-like toxin [6]. The exact role in the bacillus is unknown [6]. However, it is speculated to offer predatory protection from eukaryotic microorganisms [6]. Currently, 5 variants of mycolactone has been described and is grouped into A/B, C, D, E and F [53, 54]. Mycolactone A/B which is the most virulent variant is produced by *M. ulcerans* strains of African, Japan and Malaysia origin [55]. Ulcers are therefore, the most severe and difficult to treat [55]. Mycolactone C and D are localised to strains in the pacific regions, specifically Australia and China, respectively [55]. *Mycobacterium liflandii*, a West African frog pathogen produces the "E" variants [56, 57]. Mycolactone F is synthesised by *Mycobacterium pseudoshottsii* and *Mycobacterium marinum* [55].

Mycolactone has been observed to have cytopathic effect on host cells both *in vitro* and *in vivo* [6, 7, 58]. *M. ulcerans* upon entry into the body establishes a localised niche and multiplies along with mycolactone release [49]. The host mounts an initial cell-mediated response to clear the infection [49]. However, mycolactone functions as immune modulation and immunosuppressive agent [49, 59]. Thus preventing communication and recruitment of other important immune cells to the site of trauma [49, 60, 61]. Bacillus overload and dead inflammatory cells is usually seen as closed nodule-like or painless swellings (non-ulcerative). At this early stage, infection may clear or resolve naturally but persistent production of mycolactone eventually leads to necrotic and open ulcers [46, 49, 51].

4. Mycobacteria genus

Mycobacteria species are among well-studied genus of microorganism and *M. tuberculosis* has been an exemplar [62, 63]. The ubiquitous nature of organisms in this genus has huge medical implication [64]. Over 100 species have been identified and characterised from soil and water [64]. Mycobacteria could be divided into two main categories namely, tuberculous and non-tuberculous mycobacteria (NTM) or atypical [64]. Tuberculous mycobacteria causes diseases such as pulmonary tuberculous disease and leprosy [63]. Non-tuberculous mycobacterial species include *M. ulcerans, M. avium, M. intracellularae, M. kansasii, M. xenopi, M. chelonae, M. marinum* and *M. fortuitum* [63].

5. General overview of immune response in mammals

The natural and initial response of mammals to invading pathogens, including mycobacteria is the innate immune response [65, 66]. This involves recruitment of inflammatory cells (granulocytes) to the site of infection and subsequent ingestion and disruption of the harmful agent, which then is engulfed by macrophages [67, 68]. These are necessitated by innate immune cells, hence the name cell-mediated immunity [66]. Cell-mediate response is transient (acute) and last 1 day to 2 weeks [66]. However, humoral (antibodies) response or immunity which forms after initial expose to a pathogen is long lasting [66]. In adaptive immunity, two cells play key role [66]. These are the T (T-cell) and B (B-cell) lymphocytes [66]. T-cells develop in the bone marrow and matures in the thymus, they recognises and fights viral particulates. B-cells on the other hand matures in the bone marrow and work to eliminate bacteria and viruses from the body [66].

5.1 T-cells

T-cell is divided into "helper T cell (T_h)", "cytotoxic T cell (T_c)", "natural killer T cell (NKT)" and "memory T cell (T_m)" [66]. T_h cells are responsible for activation and proliferation of cytokines. They also assist in the maturation of B cells and activation of T_c and macrophages [66]. Helper T cell is divided into Type 1 (T_h1) and Type 2 (T_h2) T-helper cells [66]. Cell-mediated response is usually aided by T_h1. Resulting in the recruitment of macrophages to an infected site for action [66]. Interferon gamma (IFNγ) and macrophages are the main effector biomarkers of T_h1 immune response [66]. T_h1 response is usually mounted against intracellular bacteria and protozoa [66]. T_h2 on the other hand aids in the activation and proliferation of B cells, and is a component of humoral immunity [66]. T_h2 cells functions to clear extracellular bacteria from the body [66]. Eosinophils basophils, and mast cells are important effector agents of T_h2 immune response [66]. Cytotoxic T cell (T_c) is responsible for the disruption and cytolysis of host cells infected by virus [66]. They also play key role in tumour and cancer immunity [66]. Natural killer T cell (NKT) also assist in B cell activation and microbial defence [66].

5.2 B-cells

B cells is a component of the white blood cells and humoral immunity [66]. B lymphocytes secrete antibodies which are critical in pathogen specific recognition and elimination [66]. These cells are essential in the production of antigen-specific immunoglobulin (Ig) which are the agents that binds to pathogens [66]. Major sites of B cells in human include the blood and the lymph nodes [66]. Spleen and tonsil are other areas B cell are be found [66]. B cells and T cells work in concert to eliminate pathogens from the body [66]. After production and maturation in the bone marrow, B cells circulate through the blood and lymphoid system. Upon encounter with a specific pathogen, binding occurs. Subsequent assistance from the T cells lead to the elimination of the invading cell from the host [66].

6. Immune profile of active BU patients, exposed and unexposed controls

Screening for cytokines and antibodies specific responses in BU patients is still a matter of intense research [59, 60, 69–75]. This is because individuals with active disease are incapable of mounting an effective specific immune response to *M. ulcerans* [63]. It is known that patients seem to have reduced expression of T_h1 cytokines [49, 69, 70]. In comparison, T_h2 response is common among active ulcerative patients and those with healed ulcers [69, 70]. The T_h2 cytokine cells include interleukin (IL) 4, IL-5, IL-6, and IL-10. Exposed household contact with no clinical symptoms also have T_h2 response [69, 70]. However, BU patients are more likely to express IL-4 and IL-10 [69, 70, 76]. T_h1 immune response is characterised by expression of IFNγ and IL-12, critical mediators for macrophages recruitments [66, 69, 70, 76]. Interestingly, previous studies have shown that histopathology of ulcerative tissue biopsy shows macrophages with acid fast bacteria overload (likely to be *M. ulcerans*) [73, 77]. Mycolactone functions to either supress or deviate immune cells that could lead to the effective clearance of *M. ulcerans* from the host [61, 78]. Therefore, first responder cytokines such as tumour necrotic factors (TNF) is downregulated. TNF is responsible for septic shock and it works in concert with IL-17 in the release of inflammation infiltrates to infected areas and induces fever [60, 79].

7. Immune profile of BU patients undergoing antibiotic treatment

BU is curable [80], but treatment could take months if not diagnosed early [80]. Like many bacterial infection, appropriate antimicrobial medications is required in killing *M. ulcerans* to wane off mycolactone production [81, 82]. Currently, 8 weeks of oral rifampicin, is the preferred antibiotic regimen in many medical centres [46, 83]. Like mycolactone, rifampicin is a polyketide, and functions to inhibit the ribonucleic acid (RNA) polymerase activity of bacteria [84]. Thus leading to the shutdown of important amino acids, protein synthesis and inhibiting the growth of the bacillus [84]. Other medications/treatment tested or used in combination with rifampicin include Streptomycin, Oral Fluoroquinolones [85], Amikacin [86], Clofazimine [87], Co-trimoxazole [87], Ofloxacin [87], Cephalosporin [87], Penicillin [87], Metronidazol [87], Minocyclin [87], dapsone [87], Phenytoin powder [88], Topical nitrogen oxides, mycobacteriophage D29 [89], clay and local heat [87]. Cytokine profile of patients undergoing antibiotic treatment have shown that there is gradual re-establishment of T_h1 immune response during the healing process [90]. These inflammatory biomarkers include IL-4, IL-7 and IL-8 [90].

8. Paradoxical reactions in BU treatment

Paradoxical reaction in the healing process has also been reported [91]. This describes a stage where instead of the ulcers healing during antibiotic treatment, it rather becomes worst [91]. The exact mechanism underlining paradoxical reaction in BU healing is poorly understood. It has been speculated that immediate restoration of cytokine response to *M. ulcerans* antigens after mycolactone wash out could be the plausible explanation.

9. BU vaccines

There is currently no specific vaccine for BU [92]. But Bacillus Calmette–Guérin (BCG) vaccine has been used to check for cross-protection in *M. ulcerans* infection in

Uganda [50]. BCG is a purified protein derivative (PPD) from *Mycobacterium bovis* [63]. It is the main vaccination regimen for TB and some non-tuberculous mycobacteria (NTM) [63, 64]. It stimulates a strong T_h1 immune response. This include IFNγ-secreting CD4+ T cell response in recipient [64]. It was observed that BCG offered a protective effect between 47 to 50% among those tested in Uganda [50, 93]. However, this protection was short-lived, the reason is unclear [50, 94]. The main protective agent in BCG vaccine is the peptide Ag85A [92]. It is a highly conserved motif and plays a critical role in cell wall synthesis [95, 96]. Ag85A homologue from *M. ulcerans* have also been screened for cross-protection in BU disease and have shown prospect [96]. *M. ulcerans* surface protein –18 kDa small heat shock protein (MUL_2232) [97] and MUL_3720 [98] have also been used in vaccine formulation against *M. ulcerans* [99]. In a murine experiment, a recombinant (r) vaccine formulation (rMUL2232 and rMUL3720) failed to protect against BU even though antibodies were present [99]. It appears that *M. ulcerans* specific antibodies fail to protect against developing overt disease [100]. Although mycolactone is the culprit in this debilitating disease [6], vaccine based on it has been thought off as a "goose chase". The reason being, mycolatone is a polyketide, a lipid-like derivative and not necessary immunogenic [92]. Animal experiment by Robert *et al* 1997 did not find mycolactone an ideal candidate for diagnosis or vaccine [58].

10. BU and host susceptibility

M. ulcerans is an environmental pathogen [64]. Several studies have reported *M. ulcerans* DNA target both in BU endemic and non-endemic regions [21]. In addition, Sero-epidemiological studies have also shown that antibodies for the immuno-dominant protein, 18 kDa shsp is present in healthy controls [100]. This has raised numerous questions and hypotheses on host genetics and susceptibility [36]. From previous reports, it appears not all those exposed to *M. ulcerans* develop overt disease [36]. Some genetic marks such as solute carrier family 11, member 1 (*SLC11A1*) [36], autophagy-related genes E3 ubiquitin-protein ligase (PARK2) and autophagy-related protein 16–1 (ATG16L1) [36] nucleotide-binding oligomerization domain-containing 2 (NOD2) have been suggested as key players in BU susceptibility [36]. If host susceptibility is at play, it could change our perception on the mode of transmission and treatment of BU.

Author details

Michael S. Avumegah
School of Chemistry and Molecular Biosciences, The University of Queensland, Brisbane, Australia

*Address all correspondence to: s.avumegah@uq.edu.au

References

[1] World Health Organization (Buruli Ulcer) [Internet]. 2018. Available from: https://www.who.int/news-room/facts-in-pictures/detail/buruli-ulcer#:~:text=Buruli%20ulcer%20is%20caused%20by,develop%20severe%20scars%20and%20deformities [Accessed: 2022-04-07]

[2] Clancey JK. Mycobacterial skin ulcers in Uganda: Description of a new Mycobacterium (Mycobacterium Buruli). The Journal of Pathology and Bacteriology. 1964;**88**:175-187

[3] Hayman J, McQueen A. The pathology of Mycobacterium ulcerans infection. Pathology. 1985;**17**(4):594-600

[4] Weir E. Buruli ulcer: The third most common mycobacterial infection. CMAJ. 2002;**166**(13):1691

[5] Matthias G, Karl-Heinz A. The chemistry and biology of mycolactones. Beilstein Journal of Organic Chemistry. 2017;**13**:1596-1660

[6] George KM, Chatterjee D, Gunawardana G, Welty D, Hayman J, Lee R, et al. Mycolactone: A polyketide toxin from Mycobacterium ulcerans required for virulence. Science. 1999;**283**(5403):854-857

[7] George KM, Pascopella L, Welty DM, Small PL. A Mycobacterium ulcerans toxin, mycolactone, causes apoptosis in guinea pig ulcers and tissue culture cells. Infection and Immunity. 2000;**68**(2):877-883

[8] van der Werf TS, Stinear T, Stienstra Y, van der Graaf WT, Small PL. Mycolactones and Mycobacterium ulcerans disease. Lancet. 2003;**362**(9389):1062-1064

[9] WHO. Distribution of Buruli Ulcer, Worldwide, 2020. 2020

[10] O'Brien DP, Jeanne I, Blasdell K, Avumegah M, Athan E. The changing epidemiology worldwide of Mycobacterium ulcerans. Epidemiology and Infection. 2018;**147**:e19. DOI: 10.1017/S0950268818002662

[11] Muelder K, Nourou A. Buruli ulcer in Benin. Lancet. 1990;**336**(8723):1109-1111

[12] Boisvert H. Skin ulcer caused by Mycobacterium ulcerans in Cameroon. II. Bacteriological study. Bulletin de la Société de Pathologie Exotique et de ses Filiales. 1977;**70**(2):125-131

[13] Ravisse P. Skin ulcer caused by Mycobacterium ulcerans in Cameroon. I. Clinical, epidemiological and histological study. Bulletin de la Societe de pathologie Exotique. 1977;**70**(2):109-124

[14] Noeske J, Kuaban C, Rondini S, Sorlin P, Ciaffi L, Mbuagbaw J, et al. Buruli ulcer disease in Cameroon rediscovered. The American Journal of Tropical Medicine and Hygiene. 2004;**70**(5):520-526

[15] van der Werf TS, van der Graaf WT, Groothuis DG, Knell AJ. Mycobacterium ulcerans infection in Ashanti region, Ghana. Transactions of the Royal Society of Tropical Medicine and Hygiene. 1989;**83**(3):410-413

[16] Bafende AE, Phanzu MD, Imposo BB. Buruli ulcer in the Democratic Republic of Congo: Epidemiology, presentation and outcome. Tropical Doctor. 2004;**34**(2):82-84

[17] Oluwasanmi JO, Solankee TF, Olurin EO, Itayemi SO, Alabi GO,

Lucas AO. Mycobacterium ulcerans (Buruli) skin ulceration in Nigeria. The American Journal of Tropical Medicine and Hygiene. 1976;**25**(1):122-128

[18] Chukwuekezie O, Ampadu E, Sopoh G, Dossou A, Tiendrebeogo A, Sadiq L, et al. Buruli ulcer, Nigeria. Emerging Infectious Diseases. 2007;**13**(5):782-783

[19] Abrahams EW. Mycobacterium Ulcerans infection in Queensland. The Medical Journal of Australia. 1964;**1**:334-335

[20] Johnson PD, Azuolas J, Lavender CJ, Wishart E, Stinear TP, Hayman JA, et al. Mycobacterium ulcerans in mosquitoes captured during outbreak of Buruli ulcer, southeastern Australia. Emerging Infectious Diseases. 2007;**13**(11):1653-1660

[21] Merritt RW, Walker ED, Small PL, Wallace JR, Johnson PD, Benbow ME, et al. Ecology and transmission of Buruli ulcer disease: A systematic review. PLoS Neglected Tropical Diseases. 2010;**4**(12):e911

[22] Marsollier L, Robert R, Aubry J, Saint Andre JP, Kouakou H, Legras P, et al. Aquatic insects as a vector for Mycobacterium ulcerans. Applied and Environmental Microbiology. 2002;**68**(9):4623-4628

[23] Marsollier L, Stinear T, Aubry J, Saint Andre JP, Robert R, Legras P, et al. Aquatic plants stimulate the growth of and biofilm formation by Mycobacterium ulcerans in axenic culture and harbor these bacteria in the environment. Applied and Environmental Microbiology. 2004;**70**(2):1097-1103

[24] Marsollier L, Severin T, Aubry J, Merritt RW, Saint Andre JP, Legras P, et al. Aquatic snails, passive hosts of Mycobacterium ulcerans. Applied and Environmental Microbiology. 2004;**70**(10):6296-6298

[25] Silva MT, Portaels F, Pedrosa J. Aquatic insects and Mycobacterium ulcerans: An association relevant to Buruli ulcer control? PLoS Medicine. 2007;**4**(2):e63

[26] Benbow ME, Williamson H, Kimbirauskas R, McIntosh MD, Kolar R, Quaye C, et al. Aquatic invertebrates as unlikely vectors of Buruli ulcer disease. Emerging Infectious Diseases. 2008;**14**(8):1247-1254

[27] Marsollier L, Aubry J, Coutanceau E, Andre JP, Small PL, Milon G, et al. Colonization of the salivary glands of Naucoris cimicoides by Mycobacterium ulcerans requires host plasmatocytes and a macrolide toxin, mycolactone. Cellular Microbiology. 2005;**7**(7):935-943

[28] Mosi L, Williamson H, Wallace JR, Merritt RW, Small PL. Persistent association of Mycobacterium ulcerans with west African predaceous insects of the family belostomatidae. Applied and Environmental Microbiology. 2008;**74**(22):7036-7042

[29] Fyfe JA, Lavender CJ, Handasyde KA, Legione AR, O'Brien CR, Stinear TP, et al. A major role for mammals in the ecology of Mycobacterium ulcerans. PLoS Neglected Tropical Diseases. 2010;**4**(8):e791

[30] Buntine J, Crofts K, World Health Organization, & Global Buruli Ulcer Initiative. Buruli ulcer: Management of Mycobacterium ulcerans disease: A manual for health care providers (No. WHO/CDS/CPE/GBUI/2001.3). World Health Organization; 2001

[31] Ablordey A, Kotlowski R, Swings J, Portaels F. PCR amplification

with primers based on IS2404 and GC-rich repeated sequence reveals polymorphism in Mycobacterium ulcerans. Journal of Clinical Microbiology. 2005;**43**(1):448-451

[32] Fukunishi Y. Histopathological findings of Buruli ulcer: Cases from Benin in West Africa. Nihon Hansenbyō Gakkai Zasshi. 2002;**71**(3):179-186

[33] Sakyi SA, Aboagye SY, Darko Otchere I, Yeboah-Manu D. Clinical and laboratory diagnosis of Buruli ulcer disease: A systematic review. Canadian Journal of Infectious Diseases and Medical Microbiology. 2016

[34] Beissner M, Herbinger KH, Bretzel G. Laboratory diagnosis of Buruli ulcer disease. Future Microbiology. 2010;**5**(3):363-370

[35] Giles-Vernick T, Owona-Ntsama J, Landier J, Eyangoh S. The puzzle of Buruli ulcer transmission, ethno-ecological history and the end of "love" in the Akonolinga district, Cameroon. Social Science & Medicine. 2015;**129**:20-27

[36] Röltgen K, Pluschke G. Buruli ulcer: History and disease burden. Buruli Ulcer. 2019:1-41

[37] Johnson PDR, Stinear T, Small PLC, Plushke G, Merritt RW, Portaels F, et al. Buruli ulcer (M-ulcerans infection): New insights, new hope for disease control. PLoS Medicine. 2005;**2**(4):282-286

[38] Debacker M, Aguiar J, Steunou C, Zinsou C, Meyers WM, Scott JT, et al. Mycobacterium ulcerans disease: Role of age and gender in incidence and morbidity. Tropical Medicine & International Health. 2004;**9**(12):1297-1304

[39] Quek TY, Henry MJ, Pasco JA, O'Brien DP, Johnson PD, Hughes A, et al. Mycobacterium ulcerans infection: Factors influencing diagnostic delay. The Medical Journal of Australia. 2007;**187**(10):561-563

[40] O'Brien DP, Walton A, Hughes AJ, Friedman ND, McDonald A, Callan P, et al. Risk factors for recurrent Mycobacterium ulcerans disease after exclusive surgical treatment in an Australian cohort. The Medical Journal of Australia. 2013;**198**(8):436-439

[41] Loftus MJ, Tay EL, Globan M, Lavender CJ, Crouch SR, Johnson PDR, et al. Epidemiology of Buruli ulcer infections, Victoria, Australia, 2011-2016. Emerging Infectious Diseases. 2018;**24**(11):1988-1997

[42] O'Brien DP, Friedman ND, Cowan R, Pollard J, McDonald A, Callan P, et al. Mycobacterium ulcerans in the elderly: More severe disease and suboptimal outcomes. PLoS Neglected Tropical Diseases. 2015;**9**(12):e0004253

[43] O'Brien DP, Wynne JW, Buultjens AH, Michalski WP, Stinear TP, Friedman ND, et al. Exposure risk for infection and lack of human-to-human transmission of Mycobacterium ulcerans disease, Australia. Emerging Infectious Diseases. 2017;**23**(5):837-840

[44] Trubiano JA, Lavender CJ, Fyfe JA, Bittmann S, Johnson PD. The incubation period of Buruli ulcer (Mycobacterium ulcerans infection). PLoS Neglected Tropical Diseases. 2013;**7**(10):e2463

[45] Hayman J. Clinical features of Mycobacterium ulcerans infection. The Australasian Journal of Dermatology. 1985;**26**(2):67-73

[46] WHO. Laboratory Diagnosis of Buruli Ulcer Disease. 2014

[47] Tai AYC, Athan E, Friedman ND, Hughes A, Walton A, O'Brien DP.

Increased severity and spread of Mycobacterium ulcerans, Southeastern Australia. Emerging Infectious Diseases. 2018;**24**(1):58-64

[48] Roltgen K, Pluschke G. Epidemiology and disease burden of Buruli ulcer: A review. Research and Reports in Tropical Medicine. 2015;**6**:59-73

[49] Rook GA. The immunological consequences of antigen overload in experimental mycobacterial infections of mice. Clinical and Experimental Immunology. 1975;**19**(1):167-177

[50] Group UB. BCG vaccination against mycobacterium ulcerans infection (Buruli ulcer). First results of a trial in Uganda. Lancet. 1969;**1**(7586):111-115

[51] Rook GA, Carswell JW, Stanford JL. Preliminary evidence for the trapping of antigen-specific lymphocytes in the lymphoid tissue of 'anergic' tuberculosis patients. Clinical and Experimental Immunology. 1976;**26**(1):129-132

[52] Shield MJ, Stanford JL, Paul RC, Carswell JW. Multiple skin testing of tuberculosis patients with a range of new tuberculins, and a comparison with leprosy and Mycobacterium ulcerans infection. Epidemiology & Infection. 1977;**78**(3):331-348

[53] Ranger BS, Mahrous EA, Mosi L, Adusumilli S, Lee RE, Colorni A, et al. Globally distributed mycobacterial fish pathogens produce a novel plasmid-encoded toxic macrolide, mycolactone F. Infection and Immunity. 2006;**74**(11):6037-6045

[54] Kishi Y. Chemistry of mycolactones, the causative toxins of Buruli ulcer. Proceedings of the National Academy of Sciences of the United States of America. 2011;**108**(17):6703-6708

[55] Pidot SJ, Hong H, Seemann T, Porter JL, Yip MJ, Men A, et al. Deciphering the genetic basis for polyketide variation among mycobacteria producing mycolactones. BMC Genomics. 2008;**9**(1):1-15

[56] Trott KA, Stacy BA, Lifland BD, Diggs HE, Harland RM, Khokha MK, et al. Characterization of a Mycobacterium ulcerans-like infection in a colony of African tropical clawed frogs (Xenopus tropicalis). Comparative Medicine. 2004;**54**(3):309-317

[57] Tobias NJ, Doig KD, Medema MH, Chen H, Haring V, Moore R, et al. Complete genome sequence of the frog pathogen Mycobacterium ulcerans ecovar Liflandii. Journal of Bacteriology. 2013;**195**(3):556-564

[58] Roberts B, Hirst RG. Diagnostic potential of a serological assay for the diagnosis of ulcerans disease based on the putative Mycobacterium ulcerans toxin. Journal of Medical Microbiology. 1997;**46**(4):333-339

[59] Coutanceau E, Decalf J, Martino A, Babon A, Winter N, Cole ST, et al. Selective suppression of dendritic cell functions by Mycobacterium ulcerans toxin mycolactone. The Journal of Experimental Medicine. 2007;**204**(6):1395-1403

[60] Pahlevan AA, Wright DJ, Andrews C, George KM, Small PL, Foxwell BM. The inhibitory action of Mycobacterium ulcerans soluble factor on monocyte/T cell cytokine production and NF-kappa B function. Journal of Immunology. 1999;**163**(7):3928-3935

[61] Coutanceau E, Marsollier L, Brosch R, Perret E, Goossens P, Tanguy M, et al. Modulation of the host immune response by a transient intracellular stage of Mycobacterium

ulcerans: The contribution of endogenous mycolactone toxin. Cellular Microbiology. 2005;7(8):1187-1196

[62] Beer V, Bonifas V. Mycobacteria. Schweizerische Medizinische Wochenschrift. 1975;**105**(31):984-987

[63] Barksdale L, Kim SK. Mycobaterium. Bacteriological Reviews. 1977;**41**(1):217-372

[64] Kazda J, Pavlik I, Falkinham III JO, Hruska K. The Ecology of Mycobacteria: Impact on Animal's and Human's Health. Springer Science+ Business Media BV; 2009

[65] Rastogi N, Legrand E, Sola C. The mycobacteria: An introduction to nomenclature and pathogenesis. Revue Scientifique et Technique. 2001;**20**(1):21-54

[66] Riley E, Franks SA. Immunology and Evolution of Infectious Disease. Princeton University Press; 2002, 2006. p. 360. Hardback US 85.00,paperbackUS 37.95. ISBN 0 691 09595 7

[67] Connor DH, Lunn HF. Mycobacterium ulcerans infection (with comments on pathogenesis). International Journal of Leprosy. 1965;**33**(Suppl. 3):698-709

[68] Arango Duque G, Descoteaux A. Macrophage cytokines: Involvement in immunity and infectious diseases. Frontiers in Immunology. 2014;**5**:491

[69] Gooding TM, Johnson PD, Smith M, Kemp AS, Robins-Browne RM. Cytokine profiles of patients infected with Mycobacterium ulcerans and unaffected household contacts. Infection and Immunity. 2002;**70**(10):5562-5567

[70] Gooding TM, Kemp AS, Robins-Browne RM, Smith M, Johnson PD. Acquired T-helper 1 lymphocyte anergy following infection with Mycobacterium ulcerans. Clinical Infectious Diseases. 2003;**36**(8):1076-1077

[71] Prevot G, Bourreau E, Pascalis H, Pradinaud R, Tanghe A, Huygen K, et al. Differential production of systemic and intralesional gamma interferon and interleukin-10 in nodular and ulcerative forms of Buruli disease. Infection and Immunity. 2004;**72**(2):958-965

[72] Westenbrink BD, Stienstra Y, Huitema MG, Thompson WA, Klutse EO, Ampadu EO, et al. Cytokine responses to stimulation of whole blood from patients with Buruli ulcer disease in Ghana. Clinical and Diagnostic Laboratory Immunology. 2005;**12**(1):125-129

[73] Kiszewski AE, Becerril E, Aguilar LD, Kader IT, Myers W, Portaels F, et al. The local immune response in ulcerative lesions of Buruli disease. Clinical and Experimental Immunology. 2006;**143**(3):445-451

[74] Phillips R, Horsfield C, Kuijper S, Sarfo SF, Obeng-Baah J, Etuaful S, et al. Cytokine response to antigen stimulation of whole blood from patients with Mycobacterium ulcerans disease compared to that from patients with tuberculosis. Clinical and Vaccine Immunology. 2006;**13**(2):253-257

[75] Peduzzi E, Groeper C, Schutte D, Zajac P, Rondini S, Mensah-Quainoo E, et al. Local activation of the innate immune system in Buruli ulcer lesions. The Journal of Investigative Dermatology. 2007;**127**(3):638-645

[76] Zavattaro E, Mesturini R, Dossou A, Melensi M, Johnson RC, Sopoh G, et al. Serum cytokine profile during Mycobacterium ulcerans infection

(Buruli ulcer). International Journal of Dermatology. 2010;**49**(11):1297-1302

[77] Torrado E, Fraga AG, Logarinho E, Martins TG, Carmona JA, Gama JB, et al. IFN-gamma-dependent activation of macrophages during experimental infections by Mycobacterium ulcerans is impaired by the toxin mycolactone. Journal of Immunology. 2010;**184**(2):947-955

[78] Phillips R, Sarfo FS, Guenin-Mace L, Decalf J, Wansbrough-Jones M, Albert ML, et al. Immunosuppressive signature of cutaneous Mycobacterium ulcerans infection in the peripheral blood of patients with Buruli ulcer disease. The Journal of Infectious Diseases. 2009;**200**(11):1675-1684

[79] Yeboah-Manu D, Peduzzi E, Mensah-Quainoo E, Asante-Poku A, Ofori-Adjei D, Pluschke G, et al. Systemic suppression of interferon-gamma responses in Buruli ulcer patients resolves after surgical excision of the lesions caused by the extracellular pathogen Mycobacterium ulcerans. Journal of Leukocyte Biology. 2006;**79**(6):1150-1156

[80] Yotsu RR, Murase C, Sugawara M, Suzuki K, Nakanaga K, Ishii N, et al. Revisiting Buruli ulcer. The Journal of Dermatology. 2015;**42**(11):1033-1041

[81] Dega H, Robert J, Bonnafous P, Jarlier V, Grosset J. Activities of several antimicrobials against Mycobacterium ulcerans infection in mice. Antimicrobial Agents and Chemotherapy. 2000;**44**(9): 2367-2372

[82] Owusu E, Newman MJ, Addo KK, Addo P. In vitro susceptibility of Mycobacterium ulcerans isolates to selected antimicrobials. Canadian Journal of Infectious Diseases and Medical Microbiology. 2017;**2017**:5180984

[83] Phillips RO, Sarfo FS, Landier J, Oldenburg R, Frimpong M, Wansbrough-Jones M, et al. Combined inflammatory and metabolic defects reflected by reduced serum protein levels in patients with Buruli ulcer disease. PLoS Neglected Tropical Diseases. 2014;**8**(4):e2786

[84] Campbell EA, Korzheva N, Mustaev A, Murakami K, Nair S, Goldfarb A, et al. Structural mechanism for rifampicin inhibition of bacterial RNA polymerase. Cell. 2001;**104**(6):901-912

[85] O'Brien DP, McDonald A, Callan P, Robson M, Friedman ND, Hughes A, et al. Successful outcomes with oral fluoroquinolones combined with rifampicin in the treatment of Mycobacterium ulcerans: An observational cohort study. PLoS Neglected Tropical Diseases. 2012;**6**(1):e1473

[86] Marsollier L, Prevot G, Honore N, Legras P, Manceau AL, Payan C, et al. Susceptibility of *Mycobacterium ulcerans* to a combination of amikacin/rifampicin. International Journal of Antimicrobial Agents. 2003;**22**(6):562-566

[87] Sizaire V, Nackers F, Comte E, Portaels F. Mycobacterium ulcerans infection: Control, diagnosis, and treatment. The Lancet Infectious Diseases. 2006;**6**(5):288-296

[88] Adjei O, Evans MR, Asiedu A. Phenytoin in the treatment of Buruli ulcer. Transactions of the Royal Society of Tropical Medicine and Hygiene. 1998;**92**(1):108-109

[89] Trigo G, Martins TG, Fraga AG, Longatto-Filho A, Castro AG, Azeredo J, et al. Phage therapy is effective against infection by Mycobacterium ulcerans in

a murine footpad model. PLoS Neglected Tropical Diseases. 2013;7(4):e2183

[90] Martins TG, Gama JB, Fraga AG, Saraiva M, Silva MT, Castro AG, et al. Local and regional Re-establishment of cellular immunity during curative Antibiotherapy of murine Mycobacterium ulcerans infection. PLoS One. 2012;7(2)

[91] Barogui YT, Klis SA, Johnson RC, Phillips RO, van der Veer E, van Diemen C, et al. Genetic susceptibility and predictors of paradoxical reactions in Buruli ulcer. PLoS Neglected Tropical Diseases. 2016;**10**(4):e0004594

[92] Huygen K. Prospects for vaccine development against Buruli disease. Expert Review of Vaccines. 2003;**2**(4):561-569

[93] Smith PG, Revill WD, Lukwago E, Rykushin YP. The protective effect of BCG against Mycobacterium ulcerans disease: A controlled trial in an endemic area of Uganda. Transactions of the Royal Society of Tropical Medicine and Hygiene. 1976;**70**(5-6):449-457

[94] Stanford JL, Paul RC. A preliminary study of the effect of contact with environmental mycobacteria on the pattern of sensitivity to a range of new tuberculins amongst Ugandan adults. J Hyg (Lond). 1976;**76**(2):205-214

[95] Tanghe A, Content J, Van Vooren JP, Portaels F, Huygen K. Protective efficacy of a DNA vaccine encoding antigen 85A from Mycobacterium bovis BCG against Buruli ulcer. Infection and Immunity. 2001;**69**(9):5403-5411

[96] Hart BE, Hale LP, Lee S. Recombinant BCG expressing Mycobacterium ulcerans Ag85A imparts enhanced protection against experimental Buruli ulcer. PLoS Neglected Tropical Diseases. 2015;**9**(9):e0004046

[97] Diaz D, Dobeli H, Yeboah-Manu D, Mensah-Quainoo E, Friedlein A, Soder N, et al. Use of the immunodominant 18-kiloDalton small heat shock protein as a serological marker for exposure to Mycobacterium ulcerans. Clinical and Vaccine Immunology. 2006;**13**(12):1314-1321

[98] Dreyer A, Roltgen K, Dangy JP, Ruf MT, Scherr N, Bolz M, et al. Identification of the Mycobacterium ulcerans protein MUL_3720 as a promising target for the development of a diagnostic test for Buruli ulcer. PLoS Neglected Tropical Diseases. 2015;**9**(2)

[99] Bolz M, Benard A, Dreyer AM, Kerber S, Vettiger A, Oehlmann W, et al. Vaccination with the surface proteins MUL_2232 and MUL_3720 of Mycobacterium ulcerans induces antibodies but fails to provide protection against Buruli ulcer. PLoS Neglected Tropical Diseases. 2016;**10**(2):e0004431

[100] Yeboah-Manu D, Roltgen K, Opare W, Asan-Ampah K, Quenin-Fosu K, Asante-Poku A, et al. Sero-epidemiology as a tool to screen populations for exposure to Mycobacterium ulcerans. PLoS Neglected Tropical Diseases. 2012;**6**(1)

Section 3

Molecular Targets

Chapter 5

Circumsporozoite Protein from *Plasmodium vivax* and Its Relationship to Human Malaria

Luciane Moreno Storti-Melo, Gustavo Capatti Cassiano, Andrea Regina de Souza Baptista and Ricardo Luiz Dantas Machado

Abstract

The circumsporozoite surface protein (CSP) is the most abundant polypeptide in the sporozoite covering. This protein is involved in the motility and invasion of the sporozoite during its entrance in the hepatocyte. *Plasmodium vivax* CSP sequences analyses revealed that parasites have repeats belonging to three types of peptide repeat units, named VK210, VK247 or *P. vivax*-like, this last differ from the two previously described variants. All *P. vivax* CS genotypes have a worldwide distribution by genetic and serological evaluation. Studies have also reported differences in the infectivity of anophelines to the variant genotypes, indicating that different malaria vectors were more susceptible to the infection by VK210. These findings could be a consequence of differences in the emergence of this genotype in specific regions around the world. These polymorphisms are associated to the increase of nonregulated inflammatory immune responses, which in turn may be associated with the outcome of infection. Geographic coexistence of these variants increase drug resistance and also recurrent parasite behavior. Knowledge of the *P. vivax* genome contributed to several discoveries, however, new studies are still needed to evaluate its potential as a promising vaccine target.

Keywords: epidemiology, treatment response, vaccine, *plasmodium vivax*

1. Introduction

Malaria remains an important public health problem in several countries of tropical and subtropical regions of the world. In 2019, the disease caused an estimated 229 million clinical cases and around 409,000 deaths worldwide [1]. Five *Plasmodium* species are more frequently associated with human infection: Plasmodium *falciparum*, *Plasmodium vivax*, *Plasmodium malariae*, *Plasmodium ovale,* and *Plasmodium knowlesi*. The last species was recently related in a zoonotic transmission in Asia [2]. Although, cases from an outbreak in the Atlantic Forest of Rio de Janeiro state, initially diagnosed as *P. vivax* infection, were in fact caused by *Plasmodium simium*, a neotropical primate parasite [3], other simian malaria parasites, morphologically, indistinguishable from *P. vivax*, the *Plasmodium cynomolgi*, have also been shown to have the potential of zoonotic transmission to humans through the bites of infected mosquitoes under natural and experimental conditions [4, 5]. Among the natural human *Plasmodium* species causing malaria in humans, *P. vivax* is the most widely distributed and prevalent outside of Africa [6], producing more than 80 million cases per year in these regions. Once considered clinically mild when compared with *P. falciparum* infection, *P. vivax* malaria causes debilitating effects that affect social and economic indices of the endemic regions and has been associated with the occurrence of severe cases around the world.

The circumsporozoite protein (CSP) of the infective sporozoite of all *Plasmodium* species can be evidenced in the process of maturation and salivary invasion in the vector as well as in human liver cells [7, 8]. Although it has been a major target in the development of recombinant malaria vaccines, this approach had to be re-evaluated because of the discovery of sequence variation in the repetitive sequence of its central portion gene [9, 10]. All CSPs present a central repeat region (CRR) and two conserved domains RI (region I - located in the amino terminal) and RII (region II – located in the carboxyl terminal). Sequence analyses of the *P. vivax* CRR CSP showed two repeats GDRA(A/D)GQPA or ANGA(G/D)(N/D)QPG belonging to one of the nonapeptide repeat units named VK210 or VK247, respectively [11, 12]. Lately, the *P. viv*ax-like was named by Qari et al. [10] to describe an 11-mer repeat sequence, APGANQ(E/G)GGAA containing variant, distinct from the two previously described, isolated from an infected individual in Papua New Guinea (**Figure 1**, [10, 13]). However, phylogenetic analyses of the SSU RNAr and Cyt B markers positioned both *P. vivax* CS genotypes in the same clade after revealing high similarity and diversity equal to zero between VK210 and *P. vivax*-like [14].

Finally, a high frequency of IgG antibodies against the N- and C-terminal regions of the *P. vivax* CSP was detected in comparison to the immune response to the VK210- and VK247-repetitive regions. Such difference was even more pronounced in *P. vivax*-like variant-caused infection cases. So, it appears that differences among the *P. vivax* CS variants are restricted to the central repeated region of the protein, mostly generated by nucleotide variation, with important serological consequences. These are information of great importance since such genetic diversity can be the product of intra-specific biological signatures, with major implications for the *P. vivax* CSP malaria vaccine trials [14].

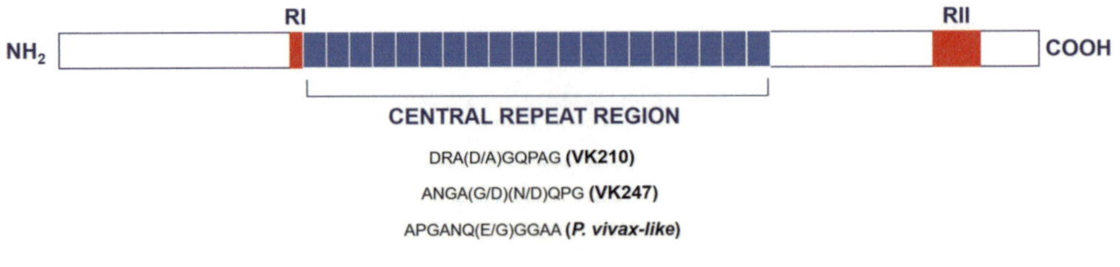

Figure 1.
Schematic representation of the circumsporozoite protein (CSP) of P. vivax*, comprising the central repeat region (CRR) flanked by the N- and C-terminal domains, including the conserved regions I and II. The CRR can have three forms denoted VK210, VK247, and* P. vivax-like*.*

2. Epidemiological aspects of the *plasmodium vivax* CSP variants in endemic areas around the world

P. vivax is responsible for approximately 7 million malaria cases worldwide [1]. In 2017, 49 countries reported locally acquired cases of *P. vivax*, where it is estimated that more than 2.5 billion people are at risk of infection [15, 16]. The control of *P. vivax* infections is more challenging compared with *P. falciparum* due to some unique biological features, such as the existence of dormant liver forms (hypnozoites) and early sexual parasite development. Thus, treatment of blood-stage infection is less effective to reduce *P. vivax* transmission, and probably the vaccine development against this species will be indispensable for elimination and eradication of disease. Most efforts to develop a vaccine against *P. vivax* have focused on the CSP. For this reason, it is important to evaluate polymorphisms in *pvcsp* gene and how its variants are widespread in endemic areas [17].

Seroepidemiological and genetic studies performed in malaria endemic areas could provide valuable information on parasite transmission and dispersion. The genetic diversity of the *CS* gene has been useful in molecular epidemiological studies, understanding the transmission, dynamics, and evolutionary relationships [14]. Furthermore, eco-epidemiological conditions, biological and genetic characteristics of the parasite, the host immunity, and local vectors may influence the different patterns of demographic expansion. On the other hand, the human intervention can become a factor to reduce the risk of malaria, without necessarily modifying the environment [18]. Serologic surveys in *P. vivax* isolates from Thailand [19, 20] and Myanmar [21] demonstrated the presence of antibodies that recognize recombinant and synthetic polypeptides that represent the VK210 and VK247 (alone or mixed). PvCSP antibodies in high-risk malaria areas in Korea [22] and sub-Saharan Africa [23] were detected. The Korean findings suggest that antibody levels for the CSP antigen could become deficient or reduced over the long-term incubation period. Mexican [24, 25] and Peruvian [24] sera reacted with either VK210 or VK247 repeat domains. It has been shown that the prevalent phenotype of the *P. vivax* parasite in the study sites of Colombia is VK247, whereas VK210 accounts for one-third of the cases, and few *P. vivax* malaria cases correspond to mixed infection [26]. Antibodies to these three variants have been circulating in the Brazilian Amazon population [27–30]. In addition, Oliveira-Ferreira et al. [31] have observed the profile of IgG responders to these PvCSP variants, where more responders to VK210 were found, followed by *P. vivax*-like and VK247 in Rondônia state. Cross-sectional cohort study included individuals from three different communities with malaria transmission in Acre state, demonstrating that VK210 presented the highest prevalence of responders to IgG antibodies, followed by *P. vivax*-like and VK247 [32]. Besides, the higher frequency of antibodies to VK210 is according to studies that described this variant as the most common in Amazon, while VK247 was rarely reported as a single infection [14, 27]. However, unlike previous reports from different areas of the Brazilian Amazon, the VK247 variant was found in higher frequencies than VK210 in Goianésia do Pará, Para State [29]. The higher frequencies of VK247 in current infections compared with higher antibody responses to VK210 may suggest that VK210 protein is more immunogenic than VK247 [33, 34], and also that the VK210 variant could have been more prevalent in endemic area from Amazon region in the recent past, as the majority of the patients had a previous history of malaria infections. Nevertheless, nucleic-acid-based diagnosis evaluates the genotypes of the current infection while antibody-based techniques are able to signalize positive results several months and even years after the end of the infection. Furthermore, there is a possibility that hypnozoites/relapses do influence the antibody response to sporozoites, since the presence of a blood-stage infection may not necessarily indicate a new infection [29, 34].

Using DNA techniques, the VK210 and VK247 sequences were found in *P. vivax* isolates from Philippines [35] and Cambodia/Thailand [36]. The cosmopolitan variant VK210 also predominate in Sri Lanka [37], Myanmar [38], Iran [39], Vanuatu Island [40], and China [41]. VK247 seems to be more common in South-eastern Asia [42, 43]. In fact, VK210 and VK247 genotypes have a worldwide distribution; however, the *P. vivax*-like genotype has been only detected in Papua New Guinea, Brazil, Indonesia, and Madagascar [13, 42, 44]. Sequence analysis of the C-terminal nonrepeat region of Myanmar VK210 variants revealed 27 distinct haplotypes. The sequence of haplotype 22 was identical with Sal I (GU339059) and accounted for 9.8% of all the VK210 sequences. The C-terminal nonrepeat region of VK247 variants showed a lower level of genetic diversity than that of VK210 variants [45]. Moreover, *pvcsp* sequencing for samples collected in Oman displayed the VK210 type with a single haplotype (six repeats of GDRADGQPA and nine repeats of GDRAAGQPA), and the malaria vector in Oman is *Anopheles culicifacies* [46]. VK210 and VK247 ratio in China was extensively investigated in several provinces, and the coexistence was verified only in Yunnan, Hainan, and Liaoning provinces, whereas in Anhui, Hubei, Guangxi, Guangdong, Guizhou, Sichuan, Jiangsu, also endemic, only the VK210 type was detected. *P. viv*ax was transmitted by distinct *Anopheline* species in China, in Henan by *An. Sinensis,* and in Hainan by *Anopheles dirus* and *Anopheles minimus*, but these two provinces had the same genotypes [47].

Malaria transmission currently exists in 21 countries and territories of the American continent, where 132 million people are at risk of infection [48]. In southern Mexico, VK210 and VK247 CSP phenotypes were detected and associated to the parasite infectivity to the local mosquito vectors *Anopheles pseudopuntipennis* and *Anopheles albimanus* [49, 50]. In samples of *P. vivax* from Mexico, Nicaragua, and Peru, it was observed that the genetic diversity of the *CSP* gene is restricted mainly to the central repeat domain and 3′-terminal portion [18]. This variation occurs due to changes in the type of nucleotides and number of repeats of the repeat region, and it is possible that the repeat region of VK247 is more stable than VK210. The predominance of VK247 parasites was documented on the Pacific Ocean coast of Western Colombia and in Piura, Peru [51]. *An. nuneztovari* infected with the VK210 and VK247 genotypes in Colombia, showing its importance for malaria transmission in areas with anthropic intervention [52]. *P. vivax* samples in the North, North-West, and South of Guatemala [53] and in municipalities of Honduras [54] were all of the VK210 genotype.

In Brazil, the detection of three *P. viva*x CSP genotypes has been observed in different areas from Amazon [44, 55–58], pre-Amazon [59], as single and mixed infections, and extra-Amazon region [60]. The VK210 genotype remains the most prevalent, most likely because of the great susceptibility of the *An. darlingi* vector, which is the most abundant in the country, to this variant [61]. The *P. vivax*-like genotype had a low frequency of the genotyped samples; this frequency could be due to its recent introduction into the region or due to differences in the development of this genotype in the vectors present in the area [27, 55]. Furthermore, the VK210 and VK247 were detected in *An. aquasalis* and *An. darlingi* in endemic areas of Pará State [61]. Although the VK210 genotype remains the most prevalent in Brazil, new evidence reveals a strong adaptation of the VK247 variant in southeastern Pará state, as well as the association of this genotype with high parasitemia. *An. albitarsis* has been found in a natural infection with the VK247 genotype in Goianésia do Pará [57], *Anopheles oswaldoi* in Acre State [62, 63]. Despite the association between high parasitemia and the VK247 genotype, the introduction of the VK247 and VK210 genotypes may have occurred at different times according to the endemic area [57].

3. CSP variants in *plasmodium vivax* isolates from malaria-endemic region and to profile these variants based on sensitivity to antimalarial drugs

As described above, *P. vivax* has a complex life cycle distinct with different stages between vector and host with a dormant liver stage. To achieve optimal results for *P. vivax* infections, effective clearance of both blood-stage parasites to treat the acute infection and liver-stage parasites (radical cure) to prevent relapse is required; however, the continual rise and propagation of resistance against antimalarial drugs are of great concern to successfully [64]. Despite increasing reports of resistance, chloroquine (CQ) remains highly effective for treatment of strains from temperate South American countries, some parts of Eastern Mediterranean, and parts of Southeast Asia [65]. The first evidence that *P. vivax* is developing resistance to CQ was reported in Papua New Guinea by Rieckmann et al. [66]. It is difficult to ascertain how common CQ resistance is in *P. vivax* infection, particularly as resistance does not appear to be absolute [67]. On the other hand, reduction in susceptibility to CQ was reported from Solomon Island [68], Papua New Guinea [69, 70], and India [71]. Brazilian studies also assessed the efficiency of standard supervised therapy or the *in vitro* profile of mefloquine (MQ) and CQ resistance showing failure of the treatment [72–74].

Another important issue is that the response to the treatment might possibly differ depending on the genotype of the parasite. However, the influence of these variants on drug response remains unclear. Studies conducted by Kain et al. [75] showed that the response to CQ may vary depending on the type of *P. vivax* variant, as both single VK210 and VK210/VK247 mixed infections took longer to clear when compared with single VK247 infection in Thailand. Later, two studies conducted in Brazil showed contradictory results. One demonstrates a correlation between the *P. vivax* variant and the response to CQ [56], and the other does not observe any difference in the frequency of the resistant isolates and in the IC_{50} mean for CQ or mefloquine, according to VK210 subtypes [74]. Additional studies will be necessary to enable a better understanding of whether individuals in endemic areas acquire *P. vivax* CSP variants that have preferential ability to malarial drug resistance.

4. Vaccine containing the three allelic variants of the *plasmodium vivax* circumsporozoite antigen

Immunologically, the course of infection by *Plasmodium* depends on the production of pro- and anti-inflammatory cytokines. In cases where an inflammatory pattern is prevalent, the disease tends to be more severe. Nonetheless, the upregulation of anti-inflammatory cytokine appears to occur after the increase in inflammatory cytokines, due to a regulatory mechanism, to prevent the exacerbation of inflammatory response and its deleterious effects [76, 77]. Moreover, *P. vivax* sporozoites are covered with CSP, a highly immunogenic protein, recognized mainly by B lymphocytes.

The good-responder immune profile against CS repeats of VK247 in individuals carrying the typically Amerindian HLA specificity DRB1*16 and the non-responder profile against CS repeats of VK210 in individuals carrying HLA DRB1*07 was previously determined [31]. Patients with the VK210 variant showed a regulatory cytokine profile in plasma, while those infected with the VK247 variant have a predominantly inflammatory cytokine profile and higher parasite loads, which altogether may result in more complications in infection. In other Brazilian Amazon areas (Maranhão and Pará state), the CSP polymorphism is associated with the increase of nonregulated inflammatory immune responses, which in turn may be associated with the outcome of infection [59]. In addition, Individuals with the rs16944 CC genotype in the *IL1β* gene have higher antibody levels to the CSP of *P. vivax* of VK247 and *P. vivax*-like variants [29].

The development of a vaccine with satisfactory efficacy for malaria would be an important strategy for the control of the disease, mainly because it provides a tool for the prevention of this parasitosis, with relevant aspects of the cost–benefit relation and would bring a solution that overlays the adaptive strategies of parasites and vectors. Despite the general obstacles that need to be overcome in the development of vaccines against parasitic diseases, researchers who develop vaccines against *P. vivax* face other adversities. One of them is the fact that these protozoa have the formation of hypnozoites, which can cause relapses months and even years after the primary infection [78]. In endemic areas of malaria transmission, individuals with repeated exposure to the parasite tend to develop clinical immunity to both P. falciparum and *P. vivax* malaria.

Since the central portion of CSP is highly immunogenic and the induction of a protective response in animals immunized with sporozoites and in humans has been observed in experimental models, CSPs are being investigated as candidates for a human vaccine against malaria. However, despite decades of research, a highly effective vaccine still remains elusive. To date, only one vaccine formulation against *P. falciparum* has been licensed, RTS, S, manufactured by GlaxoSmithKline (GSK), which showed limited protective efficacy in young children (approximately 36%). RTS, S is a recombinant vaccine produced in *Saccharomyces cerevisiae*, which comprises the C-terminal portion of PfCSP and repeat regions fused to the surface antigen (S) of hepatitis B virus. This vaccine may contribute substantially to the control of malaria when used in combination with other control measures, especially in high-risk areas [79].

This vaccine is based on CSP, the major surface antigen present in sporozoites that is critical in liver-stage development during the pre-erythrocytic life cycle [29]. CSP has a central immunodominant region of tandem repeats flanked by two highly conserved regions that encode the amino terminal and carboxy terminal regions. The most advanced vaccine candidate (phase II clinical trial) to prevent malaria by the *P. vivax* also targets CSP. Nonetheless, differently from *P. falciparum*, the PvCSP exhibits diversity in its central repetitive domain, defining the variants VK210, VK247, and *P. vivax*-like. The *P. vivax* CSP vaccine was also combined into multivalent formulations or chimeric synthetic molecules. Peptides based on the N-terminal, central repeat, and C-terminal regions of PvCSP were immunogenic in individual administrations of experimental models (mice and monkeys) as well as in healthy human volunteers [80].

Another major difficulty that must be overcome is the absence of *P. vivax* infection in rodents, and in this way, preclinical evaluations on the vaccine protective efficacy are mainly restricted to nonhuman primates. In addition to the ethical issues, these animals must undergo a surgery to remove the spleen in order to promote adequate parasitemia. This procedure may add significant result interpretation bias since organ removal causes immunological changes [81]. Thus, vaccine formulations against *P. vivax* malaria are based on chimeric parasites expressing parasite proteins [82]. The use of transgenic parasites of CSP-based vaccine formulations for the pre-erythrocytic phase of infection has allowed the analysis of functional inhibition of the exogenous CSP, expressed in replacement of the endogenous protein. Likewise, chimeric *P. berghei* parasites expressing the VK210 and VK247 were used to determine the protective efficacy of vaccine formulations consisting of viral vectors carrying *P. vivax* CSP alleles [82]. The results showed that this vaccine could induce protective and effective immune responses against P. vivax and that these findings could contribute to the development of a potential vaccine against malaria.

Another subunit vaccine against P. vivax malaria is also undergoing clinical trials. Named VMP001, this vaccine was expressed in *Escherichia coli* and encodes a chimeric CSP containing repeated sequences of the two alleles VK210 and VK247. The first Phase 1 trial with VMP001 showed that the vaccine was well tolerated and immunogenic, generating robust humoral and cellular responses to the vaccine antigen. The results did not demonstrate a protective sterilizing immunity; however, a delay to significant parasitemia was observed in more than 50% of the vaccinated individuals, compared with that seen in the control group [83].

Another study for *P. vivax* vaccine [79], which performed the expression in *Pichia pastoris* two chimeric proteins by merging the three central repeat regions of different CSP alleles (VK210, VK247, and *P. vivax*-like), after challenge with *P. berghei* ANKA transgenic parasites expressing Pb/PvVK210 or Pb/PvVK247 sporozoites. Significant time delays to parasitaemia were observed in all vaccinated mice. Thus, these formulations have potential for clinical evaluation due to their potential as protective vaccines against *P. vivax* malaria. Then, a group in Brazil describes the immunogenicity analysis of the vaccine formulations composed only by the PvCSP-AllFL chimeric and the influence of the PvAMA-1 combination [80]. The PvAMA 1 recombinant protein has also been previously described. The recombinant protein PvCSP-AllFL contains both N- and C-terminal and also the central repeats sequence of the *P. vivax* allelic variants while the central region contains six copies of the VK210 sequence (GDRA[A/D]GQPA), followed by six copies of *P. vivax*-like repeats (APGANQEGGAA) and five copies of the VK247 sequence (ANGAGNQPG). Laboratorial analyses using sporozoites from the *P. vivax* strain VK210 and blood-stage isolates demonstrated that these vaccine-elicited antibodies can recognize the native proteins. Immunization using this vaccine induced approximately a five fold decrease in parasitemia as assessed at day 5 post challenge, however, was not enough to neutralize the VK210 sporozoite infection.

5. Concluding remarks

Plasmodium vivax is the most widespread and the second most prevalent malaria-causing species in the world. CSP, although highly informative, is not a perfect measure of this parasite genetic diversity. However, this could provide interesting baseline data that allow identifying potential new cases infected by parasites diverse from those currently circulating in a determined area. Individuals residing in malaria-endemic areas may be infected with different parasite genotypes, resulting from multiple bites from infectious mosquitoes or bites from mosquitoes infected with multiple parasite genotypes. This fact can also vary considerably based on differences in the epidemiological scenarios. More investment and a greater effort toward the development of *P. vivax* vaccine components for a multispecies vaccine are required. This is due to the wide geographic coexistence of these *Plasmodium vivax* variants, but also to increased drug resistance, recent observations of severe and lethal cases of *P. vivax*, and recurrent parasite behavior. Knowledge of the *P. vivax* genome contributed to several discoveries; however, new studies to evaluate vaccines still need to be designed.

Author details

Luciane Moreno Storti-Melo[1], Gustavo Capatti Cassiano[2], Andrea Regina de Souza Baptista[3] and Ricardo Luiz Dantas Machado[3]*

1 Universidade Federal do Sergipe, São Cristovão, Sergipe, Brazil

2 Universidade de Lisboa, Lisbon, Portugal

3 Universidade Federal Fluminense, Niterói, Rio de Janeiro, Brazil

*Address all correspondence to: ricardomachado@id.uff.br

References

[1] WHO. World Health Organization. World Malaria Report. World 2019. World Health Organization. Geneva, Switzerland 2020. Available at: https://www.mmv.org/newsroom/publications/world-malaria-report-2020?gclid=Cj0KCQjwrJOMBhCZARIsAGEd4VE2kzwa9oJzJFzIr3IDdjKH5_0_w_dpxgiGSWR21oV30d4-22MVQ4caAuLREALw_wcB. Accessed on: 11-11-2021

[2] Cox-Singh J. Zoonotic malaria: *Plasmodium knowlesi*, an emerging pathogen. Current Opinion in Infectious Diseases. 2012;**25**(5):530-536

[3] Brasil P, Zalis MG, de Pina-Costa A, Siqueira AM, Júnior CB, Silva S, et al. Outbreak of human malaria caused by *plasmodium Simium* in the Atlantic Forest in Rio De Janeiro: A molecular epidemiological investigation. The Lancet Global Health. 2017;**5**(10):1038-1046

[4] Singh B, Kim SL, Matusop A, Radhakrishnan A, Shamsul SS, Cox-Singh J, et al. A large focus of naturally acquired *plasmodium knowlesi* infections in human beings. Lancet. 2004;**363**:1017-1024

[5] Ta TH, Hisam S, Lanza M, Jiram AI, Ismail N, Rubio JM. First case of a naturally acquired human infection with *plasmodium cynomolgi*. Malaria Journal. 2014;**13**:68

[6] Dalrymple U, Mappin B, Gething PW. Malaria mapping: Understanding the global endemicity of falciparum and vivax malaria. BMC Medicine. 2015;**13**:140

[7] Coppi A, Natarajan R, Pradeln G, Bennett BL, James ER, Roggero MA, et al. The malaria circumsporozoite protein has two functional domains, each with distinct roles as sporozoites journey from mosquito to mammalian host. The Journal of Experimental Medicine. 2011;**208**:341-356

[8] Suphavilai C, Looareesuwan S, Good MF. Analysis of circunsporozoite protein specific immune responses following recent infection with plasmodium vivax. The American Journal of Tropical Medicine and Hygiene. 2004;**71**:29-39

[9] Gopinath R, Wongsrichanalai C, Cordón-Rosales C, Mirrabelli L, Kyle D, Kain KC. Failure to detect a *Plasmodium vivax*-like malaria parasite in globally collected blood samples. Journal of Infectious Diseases. 1994;**170**:1630-1633

[10] Qari SH, Shi YP, Goldman IF, Udhavakumar V, Alpers MP, Collins WE, et al. Identification of *plasmodium vivax*-like human malaria parasite. Lancet. 1993a;**341**:780-783

[11] Arnot DE, Barnwell JW, Tam JP, Nussenzweig V, Nussenzweig RS. Circumsporozoite protein of *plasmodium vivax*: Gene cloning and characterization of the immunodominant epitope. Science. 1985;**230**:815-817

[12] Rosenberg R, Wirtz RA, Lanar DE, Sattabongkot J, Hall T, Waters AP, et al. Circumsporozoite protein heterogeneity in the human malaria parasite *plasmodium vivax*. Science. 1989;**245**:973-976

[13] Qari SH, Shi YP, Póvoa MM, Alpers MP, Deloron P, Murphy GS, et al. Global occurrence of *plasmodium vivax*-like human malaria parasite. The Journal of Infectious Diseases. 1993b;**168**:1485-1489

[14] Souza-Neiras WC, Storti-Melo LM, Cassiano GC, Couto VS, Couto AA, Soares IS, et al. *Plasmodium vivax* circumsporozoite genotypes: A limited variation or newsubspecies with major biological consequences? Malaria Journal. 2010;**9**:178

[15] Price RN, Commons RJ, Battle KE, Thriemer K, Mendis K. *Plasmodium vivax* in the era of the shrinking P. falciparum map. Trends in Parasitology. 2020;**36**(6):560-570

[16] Silva-Nunes M et al. Amazonian malaria: Asymptomatic human reservoirs, diagnostic challenges, environmentally driven changes in mosquito vector populations, and the mandate for sustainable control strategies. Acta Tropica. 2012;**121**(3):281-291

[17] Santamaría AM, Vásquez V, Rigg C, Samudio F, Moreno D, Romero L, et al. *Plasmodium vivax* genetic diversity in Panama: Challenges for malaria elimination in Mesoamerica. Pathogens. 2021;**10**(8):989

[18] González-Cerón L, Martinez-Barnetche J, Montero Solis C, Santillán F, Soto AM, Rodriguez MH, et al. Molecular epidemiology of *plasmodium vivax* in Latin America: Polymorphism and evolutionary relationships of the circumsporozoite gene. Malaria J. 2013;**12**(243):1-19

[19] Suwanabun N, Sattabongkot J, Wirtz RA, Rosenberg R. The epidemiology of *plasmodium vivax* circumsporozoite protein polymorphs in Thailand. The American Journal of Tropical Medicine and Hygiene. 1994;**50**(4):460-464

[20] Wirtz RA, Rosenberg R, Sattabongkot J, Webster HK. Prevalence of antibody to heterologous circumsporozoite protein of *plasmodium vivax* in Thailand. Lancet. 1990;**336**(8715):593-595

[21] Kim TS, Kim HH, Lee SS, Na BK, Lin K, Cho SH, et al. Prevalence of plasmodium vivax VK210 and VK247 subtype in Myanmar. Malaria Journal. 2010;**9**:195

[22] Lee J, Jin K, Ahn SK, Lee SK, Kwon HW, Na BK, et al. Seroprevalence of *plasmodium vivax* Circumsporozoite protein antibody in high-risk malaria areas in Korea. The Korean Journal of Parasitology. 2021;**59**(4):415-419

[23] Bwire R, Slootman EJ, Verhave JP, Bruins J, Docters van Leeuwen WM. Malaria anticircumsporozoite antibodies in Dutch soldiers returning from sub-Saharan Africa. Tropical Medicine & International Health. 1998;**3**(1):66-69

[24] Kain KC, Wirtz RA, Fernandez I, Franke ED, Rodriguez MH, Lanar DE. Serologic and genetic characterization of *plasmodium vivax* from whole blood-impregnated filter paper discs. The American Journal of Tropical Medicine and Hygiene. 1992;**46**(4):473-479

[25] Rodriguez MH, Gonzalez-Ceron L, Hernandez JE, Nettel JA, Villarreal C, Kain KC, et al. Different prevalences of *Plasmodium vivax* phenotypes VK210 and VK247 associated with the distribution of *Anopheles albimanus* and *Anopheles pseudopunctipennis* in Mexico. American Journal of Tropical Medicine and Hygiene. 2000;**62**(1):122-127

[26] Gonzalez JM, Hurtado S, Arévalo-Herrera M, Herrera S. Variants of the *plasmodium vivax* circumsporozoite protein (VK210 and VK247) in Colombian isolates. Memórias do Instituto Oswaldo Cruz. 2001;**96**:709-712

[27] Arruda ME, Zimmerman RH, Souza RM, Oliveira-Ferreira J. Prevalence and level of antibodies to the circumsporozoite protein of human malaria parasites in five states of the Amazon region of Brazil. Memórias do Instituto Oswaldo Cruz. 2007;**102**:367-371

[28] Assis GMP, de Alvarenga DAM, Costa Pereira MO, Sánchez-Arcila JC, de Pina Costa A, de Souza Junior JC, et al. Profiling humoral immune response against pre-Erythrocytic and Erythrocytic antigens of malaria parasites among Neotropical Primates in the Brazilian Atlantic Forest. Frontiers in Cellular and Infection Microbiology. 2021;**11**:678996

[29] Capobianco MP, Cassiano GC, Storti-Melo LM, Pimenta TS, Rodrigues APD, Arruda JEG, et al. Polymorphism in the IL-1β promoter is associated with IgG antibody response to circumsporozoite protein repeats of *Plasmodium vivax*. Transactions of the Royal Society of Tropical Medicine and Hygiene. 2020;**114**(11):858-865

[30] Pereira VA, Sánchez-Arcila JC, Vasconcelos MPA, Ferreira AR, de Souza Videira L, Teva A, et al. Evaluating seroprevalence to circumsporozoite protein to estimate exposure to three species of *plasmodium* in the Brazilian Amazon. Infectious Diseases of Poverty. 2018;7(1):46

[31] Oliveira-Ferreira J, Pratt-Riccio LR, Arruda M, Santos F, Daniel Ribeiro CT, Goldberg AC, et al. HLA class II and antibody responses to circumsporozoite protein repeats of *P. vivax* (VK210, VK247 and *P. vivax*-like) in individuals naturally exposed to malaria. Acta Tropica. 2004;**92**(1):63-69

[32] Soares IF, López-Camacho C, Rodrigues-da-Silva RN, da Silva MA, de Oliveira Baptista B, Totino PRR, et al. Recombinant *plasmodium vivax* circumsporozoite surface protein allelic variants: Antibody recognition by individuals from three communities in the Brazilian Amazon. Scientific Reports. 2020;**10**(1):14020

[33] Arévalo-Herrera M, Roggero MA, Gonzalez JM, Vergara J, Corradin G, López JA, et al. Mapping and comparison of the B-cell epitopes recognized on the *plasmodium vivax* circumsporozoite protein by immune Colombians and immunized *Aotus monkeys*. Annals of Tropical Medicine and Parasitology. 1998;**92**(5):539-551

[34] Céspedes N, Arévalo-Herrera M, Felger I, Reed S, Kajava AV, Corradin G, et al. Antigenicity and immunogenicity of a novel chimeric peptide antigen based on the P. vivax circumsporozoite protein. Vaccine. 2013;**31**(42):4923-4930

[35] Mann VH, Huang T, Cheng Q, Saul A. Sequence variation in the circumsporozoite protein gene of *Plasmodium vivax* appears to be regionally biased. Molecular and Biochemical Parasitology. 1994;**68**(1):45-52

[36] Sattabongkot J, Suwanabun N, Rongnoparut P, Wirtz RA, Kain KC, Rosenberg R. Comparative test of DNA probes for detection of *plasmodium vivax* circumsporozoite protein polymorphs VK247 and VK210. The Journal of Infectious Diseases. 1994;**169**(2):464-466. DOI: 10.1093/infdis/169.2.464. PMID: 8106786

[37] Dias S, Wickramarachchi T, Sahabandu I, Escalante AA, Udagama PV. Population genetic structure of the *plasmodium vivax* circumsporozoite protein (Pvcsp) in Sri Lanka. Gene. 2013;**518**:381-387

[38] Moon SU, Lee HW, Kim JY, Na BK, Cho SH, Lin K, et al. High frequency of genetic diversity of *plasmodium vivax* field isolates in Myanmar. Acta Tropica. 2009;**109**:30-36

[39] Shabani SH, Zakeri S, Mehrizi AA, Mortazavi Y, Djadid ND. Population genetics structure of *plasmodium vivax* circumsporozoite protein during the elimination process in low and unstable malaria transmission areas, southeast of Iran. Acta Tropica. 2016;**160**:23-34

[40] Chan CW, Sakihama N, Tachibana S-II, Idris ZM, Lum JK, Tanabe K, et al. *Plasmodium vivax* and *plasmodium falciparum* at the crossroads of exchange among islands in Vanuatu: Implications for malaria elimination strategies. PLoS One. 2015;**10**:e0119475

[41] Ling Zhang L, Nong Yao L, Liang Chen H, Yi Lu Q, Ruan W. Genetic diversity analysis of PvCSP and its application in tracking of *plasmodium vivax*. Experimental Parasitology. 2018;**188**:26-35

[42] Parobek CM, Bailey JA, Hathaway NJ, Socheat D, Rogers WO, Juliano JJ. Differing patterns of selection and geospatial genetic diversity within two leading *plasmodium vivax* candidate vaccine antigens. PLoS Neglected Tropical Diseases. 2014;**8**:e2796

[43] Zakeri S, Raeisi A, Afsharpad M, Kakar Q, Ghasemi F, Atta H, et al. Molecular characterization of *plasmodium vivax* clinical isolates in Pakistan and Iran using pvmsp-1, pvmsp-3α and pvcsp genes as molecular markers. Parasitology International. 2010;**59**:15-21

[44] Storti-Melo LM, de Souza-Neiras WC, Cassiano GC, Joazeiro AC, Fontes CJ, Bonini-Domingos CR, et al. *Plasmodium vivax* circumsporozoite variants and Duffy blood group genotypes in the Brazilian Amazon region. Transactions of the Royal Society of Tropical Medicine and Hygiene. 2009;**103**:672-678

[45] Võ TC, Lê HG, Kang JM, Moe M, Naw H, Myint MK, et al. Genetic polymorphism and natural selection of circumsporozoite protein in Myanmar *plasmodium vivax*. Malaria Journal. 2020;**19**(1):303

[46] Simon B, Sow F, Al Mukhaini SK, Al-Abri S, Ali OAM, Bonnot G, et al. An outbreak of locally acquired *plasmodium vivax* malaria among migrant workers in Oman. Parasite. 2017;**24**:25

[47] Liu Y, Zhou RM, Zhang YL, Wang DQ, Li SH, Yang CY, et al. Analysis of polymorphisms in the circumsporozoite protein gene of *plasmodium vivax* isolates from Henan Province. China. Malar J. 2018;**17**(1):103

[48] WHO. World Health Organization. World Malaria Report. World 2019. World Health Organization. Geneva, Switzerland 2019. Available at: https://www.mmv.org/sites/default/files/uploads/docs/publications/World%20Malaria%20Report_0.pdf. Accessed on: 5-04-2020

[49] Gonzalez-Cerón L, Rodriguez MH, Nettel JC, Villarreal C, Kain KC, Hernandez JE. Differential susceptibilities of *Anopheles albimanus* and *Anopheles pseudopunctipennis* to infections with coindigenous *plasmodium vivax* variants VK210 and VK247 in southern Mexico. Infection and Immunity. 1999;**67**:410-412

[50] Gonzalez-Cerón L, Alvarado-Delgado A, Martinez-Barnetche J, Rodriguez MH, Ovilla-Munoz M, Perez F, et al. Sequence variation of ookinete surface proteins Pvs25 and Pvs28 of *plasmodium vivax* isolates from

southern Mexico and their association to local anophelines infectivity. Infection, Genetics and Evolution. 2010;**10**:645-654

[51] Hernandez-Martinez MA, Escalante AA, Arevalo-Herrera M, Herrera S. Antigenic diversity of the *plasmodium vivax* circumsporozoite protein in parasite isolates of Western Colombia. The American Journal of Tropical Medicine and Hygiene. 2011;**84**:51-57

[52] Naranjo-Díaz N, Altamiranda M, Luckhart S, Conn JE, Correa MM. Malaria vectors in ecologically heterogeneous localities of the Colombian Pacific region. PLoS One. 2014;**9**(8):e103769

[53] Mendizábal-Cabrera R, Padilla N. Diversidad genética de Plasmodium Vivax Em Regiones de Alto Riesgo de Malaria en Guatemala [Genetic Diversity of. *Plasmodium Vivax* in Areas of High Risk of Malaria in Guatemala]. Guatemala: Revista de la Universidad del Valle de Guatemala; 2006. pp. 62-79

[54] Lopez AC, Ortiz A, Coello J, Sosa-Ochoa W, Torres RE, Banegas EI, et al. Genetic diversity of *plasmodium vivax* and *plasmodium falciparum* in Honduras. Malaria Journal. 2012;**11**:391

[55] Machado RL, Póvoa MM. Distribution of *plasmodium vivax* variants (VK210, VK247 and *P. vivax*-like) in three endemic areas of the Amazon region of Brazil and their correlation with chloroquine treatment. Transactions of the Royal Society of Tropical Medicine and Hygiene. 2000;**94**:377-381

[56] Machado RL, de Filho AF, Calvosa VSP, Figueredo MC, Nascimento JM, Póvoa MM. Correlation between *plasmodium vivax* variants in Belém, Pará state, Brazil and symptoms and clearance of parasitaemia. Brazilian J Infect Dis. 2003;**7**:175-177

[57] Santos EA, Primo DG, Sucupira IMC, Cassiano GC, Barbosa DRL, Vianna GMR, et al. Frequency of *Plasmodium vivax* circumsporozoite protein genotypes in humans and anopheline mosquitoes in an endemic area of southeastern Pará state, Brazil. Revista Pan-Amazônica de Saúde. 2016;**7**:57-64

[58] Gomes MD, Vieira JL, Cassiano GC, Musset L, Legrand E, Nacher M, et al. Evaluation of Cimcrusporozoite Protein of *Plasmodium vivax* to estimate its prevalence in Oiapoque, Amapá State, Brazil, Bordering French Guiana. Revista do Instituto de Medicina Tropical de São Paulo. 2016;**58**:72

[59] de Ribeiro BP, Cassiano GC, de Souza RM, Cysne DN, Grisotto MA, de Azevedo dos Santos AP, et al. Polymorphisms in *Plasmodium vivax* Circumsporozoite protein (CSP) influence parasite burden and cytokine balance in a pre-Amazon endemic area from Brazil. PLoS Neglected Tropical Diseases. 2016;**10**(3):e0004479

[60] Almeida-de-Oliveira NK, Abreu-Fernandes R, Lima-Cury L, Lavigne AR, Pina-Costa A, Perce-da-Silva DS, et al. Balancing selection and high genetic diversity of *plasmodium vivax* circumsporozoite central region in parasites from Brazilian Amazon and Rio de Janeiro Atlantic Forest. PLoS One. 2020;**15**(11):e0241426

[61] Silva AN, Santos CC, Lacerda RN, Machado RL, Póvoa MM. Susceptibility of *Anopheles aquasalis* and *An. darlingi* to *Plasmodium vivax* VK210 and VK247. Memórias do Instituto Oswaldo Cruz. 2006;**101**:547-550

[62] Branquinho MS, Araújo MS, Natal D, Marrelli MT, Rocha RM, Taveira FA, et al.

Anopheles oswaldoi a potential malaria vector in acre, Brazil. Transactions of the Royal Society of Tropical Medicine and Hygiene. 1996;**90**(3):233

[63] Marrelli MT, Branquinho MS, Hoffmann EH, Taipe-Lagos CB, Natal D, Kloetzel JK. Correlation between positive serology for *plasmodium vivax*-like/*plasmodium simiovale* malaria parasites in the human and anopheline populations in the state of acre, Brazil. Transactions of the Royal Society of Tropical Medicine and Hygiene. 1998;**92**(2):149-151

[64] Malaria Threats Map–Parasite Drug Resistance, 2018. World Health Organization, Geneva. Available at: http://apps.who.int/malaria/maps/threats/

[65] Woon SA, Manning L, Moore BR. Antimalarials for children with *plasmodium vivax* infection: Current status, challenges, and research priorities. Parasitology International. 2021;**13**:102512

[66] Rieckmann KH, Davis DR, Hutton DC. *Plasmodium vivax* resistance to chloroquine? Lancet. 1989;**2**(8673):1183-1184

[67] Collignon P. Chloroquine resistance in *Plasmodium vivax*. The Journal of Infectious Diseases. 1991;**164**(1):222-223

[68] Whitby M, Wood G, Veenendaal JR, Rieckmann K. Chloroquine-resistant *Plasmodium vivax*. Lancet. 1989;**2**(8676):1395

[69] Schuurkamp GJ, Spicer PE, Kereu RK, Bulungol PK, Rieckmann KH. Chloroquine-resistant *Plasmodium vivax* in Papua New Guinea. Transactions of the Royal Society of Tropical Medicine and Hygiene. 1992;**86**(2):121-122

[70] Murphy GS, Basri H, Purnomo AEM, Bangs MJ, Mount DL, Gorden J, et al. Vivax malaria resistant to treatment and prophylaxis with chloroquine. Lancet. 1993;**341**(8837):96-100

[71] Garg M, Nagnur S, Potkar CN, Kshirsagar NA. General practitioners and treatment of malaria-need for continuing medical education. Journal of the Association of Physicians of India. 1995;**43**(8):584-585

[72] de Santana Filho FS, Arcanjo AR, Chehuan YM, Costa MR, Martinez-Espinosa FE, Vieira JL, et al. Chloroquine-resistant *Plasmodium vivax,* Brazilian Amazon. Emerging Infectious Diseases. 2007;**13**(7):1125-1126

[73] Marques J, Moles E, Urbán P, Prohens R, Busquets MA, Sevrin C, et al. Application of heparin as a dual agent with antimalarial and liposome targeting activities toward plasmodium-infected red blood cells. Nanomedicine. 2014;**10**(8):1719-1728

[74] Pratt-Riccio LR, Baptista BO, Torres VR, Bianco-Junior C, Perce-Da-Silva DS, Riccio EKP, et al. Chloroquine and mefloquine resistance profiles are not related to the circumsporozoite protein (CSP) VK210 subtypes in field isolates of *Plasmodium vivax* from Manaus, Brazilian Amazon. Memórias do Instituto Oswaldo Cruz. 2019;**114**:e190054

[75] Kain KC, Brown AE, Lanar DE, Ballou WR, Webster HK. Response of *Plasmodium vivax* variants to chloroquine as determined by microscopy and quantitative polymerase chain reaction. American Journal of Tropical Medicine and Hygiene. 1993;**49**(4):478-484

[76] Andrade BB, Reis-Filho A, Souza-Neto SM, Clarêncio J, Camargo LMA, Barral A, et al. Severe

Plasmodium vivax malaria exhibits marked inflammatory imbalance. Malaria Journal. 2010;**9**:13-20

[77] Medina TS, Costa SPT, Oliveira MD, Ventura AM, Souza JM, Gomes TF, et al. Increased interleukin10 and interferon-g levels in *plasmodium vivax* malaria suggest a reciprocal regulation which is not altered by IL-10 gene promoter polymorphism. Malar J. Bio Med Central Ltd. 2011;**10**:264

[78] Gimenez AM, Salman AM, Marques RF, López-Camacho C, Harrison K, Kim YC, et al. A universal vaccine candidate against plasmodium vivax malaria confers protective immunity against the three PvCSP alleles. Scientific Reports. 2021;**11**(1):17928

[79] de Camargo TM, de Freitas EO, Gimenez AM, Lima LC, de Almeida CK, Françoso KS, et al. Prime-boost vaccination with recombinant protein and adenovirus-vector expressing *Plasmodium vivax* circumsporozoite protein (CSP) partially protects mice against Pb/Pv sporozoite challenge. Scientific Reports. 2018;**8**(1):1118

[80] Lima LC, Marques RF, Gimenez AM, Françoso KS, Aliprandini E, Camargo TM, et al. A multistage formulation based on full-length CSP and AMA-1 Ectodomain of *plasmodium vivax* induces high antibody Titers and T-cells and partially protects mice challenged with a transgenic *Plasmodium berghei* parasite. Microorganisms. 2020;**8**(6):916

[81] Yadava A, Waters NC. Rationale for further development of a vaccine based on the Circumsporozoite protein of *plasmodium vivax*. PLoS Neglected Tropical Diseases. 2017;**11**(1):e0005164

[82] Naz S, Ahmad S, Abbasi SW, Ismail S, Waseem S, Tahir Ul Qamar M, et al. Identification of immunodominant epitopes in allelic variants VK210 and VK247 of *plasmodium vivax* Circumsporozoite immunogen. Infection, Genetics and Evolution. 2021;**96**:105120

[83] Bennett JW et al. Phase 1/2a trial of *plasmodium vivax* malaria vaccine candidate VMP001/AS01B in malaria-naive adults: Safety, immunogenicity, and efficacy. PLoS Neglected Tropical Diseases. 2016;**10**:e0004423

Chapter 6

Exploring the Evolutionary Origin and Biological Role of the *Trypanosoma cruzi* Ecotin-Like Molecule in Chagas' Disease

Carla Moreira Santana, Max Mario Fuhlendorf, Felipe Baena Garcia, Edmar Silva Santos, Ângela Maria Lourenço, Cristiane Castro Faccini, Abílio Augusto Fragata Filho, Aline Diniz Cabral and Márcia Aparecida Sperança

Abstract

Enzymes called proteases play important roles in the physiology of all living organisms and in the interaction of a parasite/symbiont with its host. Different types of peptidases act on specific substrates and are regulated by specific inhibitors. Ecotins, described firstly in *Eschericchia coli*, are inhibitors of serine peptidases (ISP) from S1A family including trypsin, chymotrypsin, neutrophil elastase, and cathepsin G. Ecotin-like inhibitors are present in parasites from Trypanosomatidae family, including *Trypanosoma cruzi*, the causative agent of Chagas' disease. This chapter explores the evolutive origin of the *T. cruzi* TcISP2 and its possible interactions with proteins of the human immune system and in Chagas' disease. The phylogenetic relationship of TcISP2 with trypanosomatids ISPs, comparative loci analysis among trypanosomatids, and the occurrence of bacteria endosymbionts in the group strongly suggest horizontal transfer as the main origin mechanism for trypanosomatids ISPs, followed by duplication events and losses that could explain its current genomic pattern. The relationship of TcISP2 with the vertebrate host immune system can be inferred by its antigenicity in Chaga's disease murine model, presenting high antibody titer after 60 days post-infection, which could indicate the inhibition of TcISP2 activity associated with chronic phase of the Chaga's disease.

Keywords: *Trypanosoma cruzi*, ecotin, serine-protease inhibitor, recombinant protein, neutrophil elastase

1. Introduction

Chagas disease, despite the success of public policies for vector control, still has a worrying annual incidence in Brazil, especially in the precarious and growing frontiers of the legal Amazon [1]. The etiologic agent of Chagas' disease is the protozoan *Trypanosoma cruzi*, transmitted through the bites of insects of the Triatominae subfamily, in blood transfusions, or orally through the ingestion of contaminated food with the waste of vector insects [2]. The incidence of the disease through classical transmission by triatomines cohabiting human residences has been significantly reduced as a result of the effectiveness of public vector control and housing improvement programs [3]. However, there is a growing number of cases in the states of the Legal Amazon, where there are wild triatomines that, as they do not invade human dwellings, cannot be easily controlled by traditional containment measures [4]. The frequent result is oral contamination through ingestion of products contaminated by vectors infected with *Trypanosoma cruzi*, such as açaí pulp [5], in addition to the expansion of vector transmission by wild triatomines, whose incidence only should grow as deforestation continues in the region [6]: between 2000 and 2016, more than 2000 confirmed acute cases in Belém in the State of Pará, Brazil, Amazon region [7].

T. cruzi belongs to the order Trypanosomatida, which also harbors the genus *Leishmania*, another widely distributed human parasite that causes leishmaniasis, also, an important neglected disease. Genetic analysis of members of this order revealed the presence of genes that encode serine peptidase inhibitors (ISPs), in the genera *Leishmania* and *Trypanosoma.* The ISPs observed in these trypanosomatids are orthologs of ecotin, an inhibitor found only in gram-negative bacteria [8], suggesting a possible lateral genetic transfer at some point in the evolution of these taxa. This fact, quite interesting in itself, becomes more intriguing when we consider that the sequencing did not reveal the presence, in the genome of the studied parasites, of serine peptidases of the types that ecotin inhibits, as it indicates that trypanosomatid ISPs have exogenous targets [9].

In bacteria, especially those that invade arthropod and vertebrate tissue, a growing variety of studies indicates that ecotin is a key factor in defense against the immunological barriers of infected organisms. Recent evidence indicates that ISPs synthesized by *Leishmania major*, which are also ecotin orthologs, have an exogenous function, facilitating the parasite's survival against the host immune system. Drawing a parallel between studies with ecotin-bearing bacteria and ISPs of *L. major* —a parasite that belongs to a sister group of *T. cruzi*—it is clear the fundamental role that these serine peptidase inhibitor proteins play in modulating the immune response of these parasite hosts. Next, we compared the position of ecotin in various members of the Kinetoplastida group to reinforce the hypothesis of its possible common origin from horizontal transfer. Besides, the interaction of ISP2 from *T. cruzi* (TcISP2) with the vertebrate host immune system will be demonstrated by its antigenicity property in the murine model of Chagas' disease.

1.1 General taxonomic aspects and life cycle of *Trypanosoma cruzi*

Kinetoplastida is a class of unicellular eukaryotes characterized by the presence of the kinetoplast, a feature formed by circular concatenated DNA molecules (kDNA) inside a solitary mitochondrion [10]. Trypanosomatida is an order of kinetoplastids composed of obligatory parasites of invertebrates, plants, and all classes of vertebrates [11, 12]. This order includes genera that are exclusive arthropod parasites, such as *Crithidia* [13, 14] and *Herpetomonas* [11], and also genera with heteroxenous life cycles (involving more than one host), such as *Leishmania* and *Trypanosoma*. These two genera are of great medical importance as they contain species that are etiological agents for serious human diseases, such as sleeping sickness, Chagas' disease, and visceral and cutaneous leishmaniasis. Some Trypanosomatida genera have obligate endosymbiont bacteria, which have been used as model organisms in studies on unicellular symbiosis [15, 16].

Species in the *Trypanosoma* genus are heteroxenous and usually have complex life cycles [17]. In trypanosomatids belonging to the *Stercoraria* section, trypanosomes are transmitted to vertebrate hosts by hemipteran insects in the Reduviidae family [18], such as *Trypanosoma cruzi*, the etiological agent of Chagas' disease. Motile metacyclic trypomastigote infective form of *T. cruzi* penetrates the skin or skin lesion of the vertebrate host after being expelled with the feces of the insect. Once inside the vertebrate host, the infective metacyclic trypomastigotes transform into bloodstream trypomastigotes, which invade cells of various tissues and, differentiate into amastigotes, static forms that multiply inside the cells by binary fission. After a number of division cycles, *T. cruzi* amastigotes transform into bloodstream trypomastigotes and are released into the circulatory system, infecting other cells in the body. When a triatomine insect vector feeds on an infected vertebrate with the motile trypomastigotes present in the blood, the ingested parasite differentiates into epimastigote forms that multiply by binary fission and migrate to the posterior intestine of the insect where it transforms to vertebrate infective metacyclic trypomastigotes, completing the parasite cycle. In members of the *Salivaria* section of *Trypanosoma* genera, such as *Trypanosoma brucei*, the metacyclic trypomastigote is injected directly from the salivary gland of the insect host, flies from *Glossina* genus, into the bloodstream of the vertebrate host [19, 20]. *T brucei* trypomastigotes can directly multiply by binary fission in the vertebrate blood. When a hematophagous insect vector feeds on the blood of an infected vertebrate it consumes bloodstream trypomastigotes forms, which differentiate inside the insect into procyclic trypomastigotes and then into epimastigotes, which are capable of multiplying by binary fission. The cycle is closed with the transformation of epimastigote forms into metacyclic trypomastigote forms in the salivary gland of the insect fly that infects a new vertebrate host during blood feeding [18].

The heteroxenous life cycle in trypanosomatids may have an evolutionary history beginning before the start of the tertiary period, but the overall Kinetoplastida phylogeny is still filled with uncertainty, even more so among trypanosomatids [21]. The existence of bacterial endosymbionts in the group is of marked interest to researchers, possibly being related to the transition from free to parasitic life cycles or being involved in lateral gene transfers between bacteria and eukaryotes [22]. Trypanosomatids have polycistronic DNA transcription which tends to keep coding sequences conserved in contiguous groups, resulting in multiple gene loci being preserved between different species [23].

1.2 Serine protease inhibitors: ecotins and *Trypanosomatida* ISPs

Ecotins are serine protease inhibitors initially described in *E. coli* bacteria and named for their capacity to inhibit the digestive enzyme trypsin—*E. coli* trypsin inhibitor [8]. The *E. coli* ecotin has a molecular weight of 18 kDa and is expressed in the cellular periplasm with a homodimeric active form. It inhibits serine proteases of family S1A, including trypsin, chymotrypsin, neutrophil elastase, and cathepsin G [24, 25]. Ecotin activity protect cells against exogenous serine peptidases involved in various biological processes, including coagulation and fibrinolysis; this capacity for inhibiting a considerable number of different proteins differentiates ecotin from most other serine protease inhibitors, which generally are highly specific [26–29].

Trypanosomatids are the only eukaryotes with genes coding for ecotin analogs, described for the first time in 2005 by Ivens et al. in *L. major*, with three variants that were named ISP1, ISP2, and ISP3 [9, 30]. In *L. major*, the ISP1 and ISP2 ecotins have 16.5 and 17.5 kDa, respectively, and while structurally similar to the *E. coli* ecotin, their amino acid sequence identity is only 36% [31], and they have different patterns of expression and inhibitory activity in the various stages of the parasite life cycle [30]. In *L. major,* the ISP1 variant is expressed in larger quantities in the life cycle forms living in the insect host, and knockout studies with this gene suggest that it has endogenous functions, mainly in the flagellar formation process [31]. Also in *L. major*, ISP2 expression occurs in all life cycle stages and there are evidences that this enzyme participates in the parasite macrophage infection process in hosts, by inhibiting serine proteases such as neutrophil elastase in vertebrates. There is evidence that *Leishmania* parasites with knocked down ISP2 suffer more intense phagocytosis by host macrophages [30, 32, 33]. *E. coli* and other bacteria that have periplasmic ecotin use it to evade hosts' immune systems, and *L. major* employs its ISP2 inhibitor in a similar fashion [26, 34]. The lack of genes coding for ecotin target enzymes (the S1A family of serine proteases) in both *E. coli* and *L. major* is a strong indicator of the probable role of ecotins in these species' interactions with vertebrate hosts [30].

An ISP2 homolog has been found in *T. cruzi* with a high degree of sequence similarity to the *L. major* gene [35]. BLAST searches in the NCBI GenBank database reveal that other members of the genus *Trypanosoma* also possess ISP2 homologs, as well as close relatives in the order Trypanosomatida such as *Leptomonas* spp., most papers published on the subject have focused on *Leishmania* ISPs. It is probable that, due to both its conservation in various species of trypanosomatids and its flexible functional properties, ecotin homologs have offered some fitness gain to trypanosomatids with vertebrate hosts. Also, the conservation of ISPs in various species indicates an origin in the common ancestor of Trypanosomatida. The similarity between trypanosomatid ISPs and bacterial ecotins makes us raise the hypothesis of a lateral gene transfer between *E. coli*-like bacteria and the common ancestor of the various Trypanosomatida genera as the origin of ISPs [30, 36]. Recent research suggest that this kind of lateral gene transfer has been essential in this group's evolutionary history [22]. The bacterial endosymbionts in Kinetoplastida are in class Betaproteobacteria [37]. This group contains vertebrate infecting species that not only possess ecotin-encoding genes, but that depends on those ecotins being expressed to maintain their virulence [34], which may be another hint of ancestral lateral gene transfers between Betaproteobacteria and Trypanosomatida.

Leishmania and *Trypanosoma* parasites are responsible for a number of severely neglected tropical diseases, as officially listed by the World Health Organization [38]. Multiple sources indicate that ecotin and its homologs are connected to these parasites' infective capacity, but research in this specific subject is still timid, especially in the *Trypanosoma* genus. Neglected tropical diseases like Chagas' disease (caused *by T. cruzi*) and African sleeping sickness (caused by *T. brucei*) are neglected for socio-historical reasons, as these afflictive diseases rarely, if ever, occur in developed countries.

The evolution of the genes encoding for trypanosomatid ISPs can shed light not only on the group's evolutionary history but also on the overall importance of this enzyme for future researchers. In the next few pages, we show evidence for a common ancestry of ISPs in extant trypanosomatids using both phylogenetic inferences and a novel method for gene loci analysis. Also, we demonstrate the antigenicity of *T. cruzi* ISP2 in the murine model of Chagas' disease and the presence of a higher concentration of antibodies against TcISP2 in the chronic phase of infection.

2. Methodology

2.1 Phylogenetic methods

Amino acid sequences of ISPs were obtained from the NCBI database (*National Center for Biotechnology Information, U.S. National Library of Medicine*) using their BLAST search package using *E. coli* ecotin as a BLAST target [39]. Sequence alignment using the MUSCLE algorithm and phylogenetic maximum likelihood analysis was done in SeaView [40], with the selection of best-fit amino acid substitution matrices done with PROTTEST 3 [41]. Resulting tree files were manually edited to standardize terminal labels, and cladogram image files were exported using the iTol web tree tool (**Figure 1**) [42].

For the loci viewer project database input, complete genomic sequences for loci analysis were obtained from the same database using tBLASTn, a tool that takes amino acid sequences as input and searches for corresponding nucleotide sequences, with the search limited to RefSeq annotated genomes [39]. Data was input and manipulated into custom software developed for the author's master thesis [43]. The complete list of sequences with respective web links and NCBI GenBank IDs is listed in **Table 1**. After data input was completed, the database was manually manipulated using SQL queries to identify close genes to the left or right of the ecotin homologs in various species, aided by the visual map generated showing that ISPs occurred in two different loci around 50 kbp apart in most species. One of these genes is a putative katanin-encoding gene, and the other three are conserved hypothetical protein-encoding genes that were called CHP1, 2, and 3. Using the *L. braziliensis* genome as a reference, these four amino acid sequences were run through the NCBI tBLASTn tool using the same settings used for the ecotin homologs, and resulting CDSs were manually labeled *CHP1*, *CHP2*, *CHP3*, and *katanin-like* in the loci viewer database.

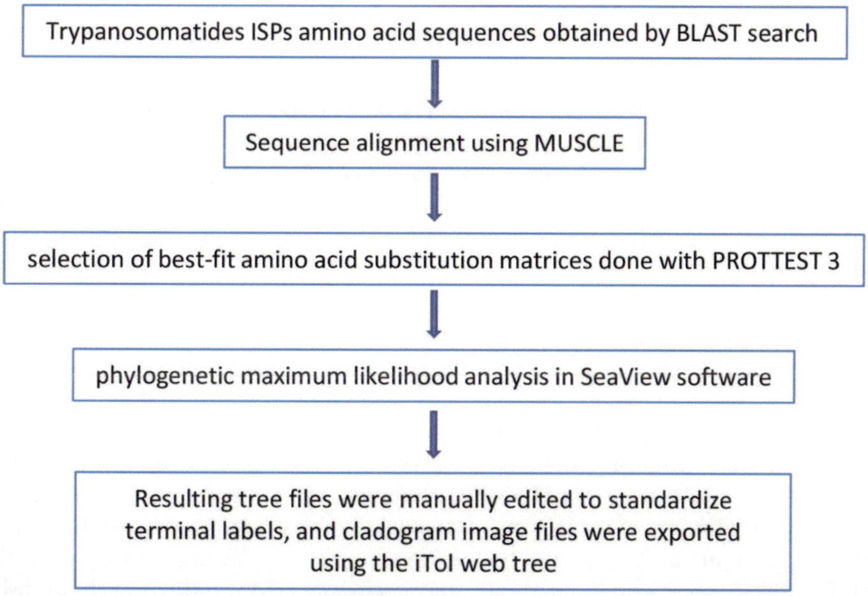

Figure 1.
Scheme on methodology employed in the phylogenetic reconstruction of ISPs from trypanosomatids.

Leishmania braziliensis MHOM/BR/75/M2904	NC_009307.2	https://www.ncbi.nlm.nih.gov/nuccore/NC_009307.2
Leishmania braziliensis MHOM/BR/75/M2904	NC_018242.1	https://www.ncbi.nlm.nih.gov/nuccore/NC_018242.1
Leishmania infantum JPCM5	NC_009399.2	https://www.ncbi.nlm.nih.gov/nuccore/NC_009399.2
Leishmania major strain Friedlin	NC_007256.2	https://www.ncbi.nlm.nih.gov/nuccore/NC_007256.2
Leishmania mexicana MHOM/GT/2001/U1103	NC_018319.1	https://www.ncbi.nlm.nih.gov/nuccore/NC_018319.1
Leishmania panamensis	NC_025860.1	https://www.ncbi.nlm.nih.gov/nuccore/NC_025860.1
Leptomonas pyrrhocoris	NW_015438382.1	https://www.ncbi.nlm.nih.gov/nuccore/NW_015438382.1
Leptomonas pyrrhocoris	NW_015438394.1	https://www.ncbi.nlm.nih.gov/nuccore/NW_015438394.1
Trypanosoma brucei TREU927	NC_007278.1	https://www.ncbi.nlm.nih.gov/nuccore/NC_007278.1
Trypanosoma brucei gambiense DAL972	NC_026738.1	https://www.ncbi.nlm.nih.gov/nuccore/NC_026738.1
Trypanosoma cruzi strain CL Brener	NW_001849489.1	https://www.ncbi.nlm.nih.gov/nuccore/NW_001849489.1
Trypanosoma grayi	NW_008825978.1	https://www.ncbi.nlm.nih.gov/nuccore/NW_008825978.1
Trypanosoma grayi	NW_008826261.1	https://www.ncbi.nlm.nih.gov/nuccore/NW_008826261.1

Table 1.
List of RefSeq genomic records inserted into the loci image generator database.

2.2 Purification of recombinant TcISP2 (TcISP2r) from *Escherichia coli*

The construction of recombinant plasmid to express TcISP2r in *E. coli* and extraction of TcISP2r were previously described by our research group [44]. Initially, a culture of *E. coli* from DH5α strain was transformed with pET28a plasmid containing TcISP2r construction with a histidine tag at N-terminus, in the presence of 50 ug/mL of Kanamycin at 600 nm optical density of 0,5, following expression induction with 1 mM of IPTG and incubation for more 16 hours in the shaker at 37°C. For protein extraction, 50 mL of bacteria culture was precipitated by centrifugation and the pellet was dissolved in 6 mL of 20 mM of phosphate buffer pH 7.4 and 0.024 g of lysozyme (Sigma, USA), and incubated at room temperature for 15 minutes. Then 6 ml of lysis buffer (20 mM phosphate buffer pH 7.4 and 0.5% Tween 20) was added and incubated for 30 minutes at 37°C. Finally, the bacterial lysate was centrifuged at 8000 x g for 15 minutes at 4°C to precipitate cell debris. The protein present in the supernatant was purified on an affinity chromatography column containing nickel, HisPur Ni-NTA Spin 0.2 ml (Thermo Fisher Scientific, USA), following the supplier's instructions. After passing the entire supernatant through the column by successive centrifugations at low speed (4000 x g) for 1 min, the column was washed with 10 volumes of 20 mM phosphate buffer pH 7.4 with 20 mM Imidazole. Subsequently, the protein was eluted from the column with 150 mM Imidazole. The purified TcISP2r protein was subjected to concentration by filtration on 10 KDa cellulose filters to replace the 20 mM phosphate buffer pH 7.4 containing 150 mM imidazole with 20 mM phosphate buffer pH 7.4 without imidazole. The final protein concentration was determined by absorbance at 280 nm in a UV light spectrophotometer. The quality and quantity of protein obtained were also verified by protein electrophoresis in 12% acrylamide gel. Protein specificity was verified by Western Blotting using an anti-histidine antibody.

2.3 Obtention of sera from murine model of acute and chronic Chagas' disease

The murine model of acute and chronic Chagas' disease is already established in the Chagas Disease laboratory of the Instituto Dante Pazzanese. For the proposed study, a total of 8 male mice, Black-C57, 20 days old, were inoculated intraperitoneally with $1x10^4$ parasites per milliliter (mL) in 0.9% saline, pH 6.0, and three animals were used as negative controls.

After infection, 200 to 400 uL of blood samples were collected from the mice on days 7, 15 (acute phase of infection), 30, 45, and 60 (chronic phase of infection) after infection, through submandibular vein puncture, and centrifuged at 1200 x g for 10 minutes at 25°C, to obtain the serum, which was stored at −20°C until analysis. On day 60, the mice were euthanized in a chamber with cotton soaked in Sevoflurane (C4H3F7O), following cervical dislocation to ensure death. After euthanasia, a necropsy of brain tissue, liver, spleen, kidneys, and heart was performed. The heart was washed with saline and cardiac tissue and saline lavage were stored at −20°C. The euthanasia method was performed according to the recommendations of the Brazilian guide to good practices for the euthanasia of animals established by the consultants of the Ethics, Bioethics and Animal Welfare Committee of the Federal Council of Veterinary Medicine (CEBEA/CFMV). All handling of the animals was carried out in accordance with the Brazilian guideline for the care and use of animals for scientific and educational purposes (DBCA), of the National Council for the Control of Animal Experimentation (CONCEA) (https://www.sbcal.org.br/download/download?ID_DOWNLOAD=58). The protocol was approved by the Animal Research Ethics Committee of the Instituto Dante Pazzanese (Registration number 020/2019).

T. cruzi infection was confirmed by reading slides containing blood smears and by polymerase chain reaction (PCR) with the oligonucleotides Tc121 (5′ AAATAATGTACGGGKGAGATGCATGA 3′) and Tc122 (5′ GGTTCGATTGGGGTTGGTGTAATATA 3′), which amplifies a 330 bp fragment corresponding to *T. cruzi* kDNA [45, 46]. The PCR reaction was performed with the enzyme Platinum Taq DNA polymerase (ThermoFischer Scientific), according to the supplier's instructions. The cycles used for amplification were 3 min 94°C/40x 94°C 1 min; 62°C 1 min; 72°C 1 min/7 min 72°C. PCR products were analyzed on 2% agarose gel stained with ethidium bromide.

2.4 Standardization of TcISP2 enzyme-linked immunosorbent assay (ELISA)

To perform the indirect ELISA test for antibodies against TcISP2r, the binding efficiency of the recombinant protein was initially verified in 96-well plates with low, medium, and high binding capacity (**Figure 2**). Each of the plaque types was sensitized with 1.0, 2.0, and 5 μg of TcISP2r protein diluted in 0.2 M

High binding

	1	2	3	4	5	6	7	8	9	10	11	12	
A	0,525	0,216	0,086	0,074	0,483	0,286	0,088	0,073	0,397	0,203	0,079	0,066	405
B	0,34	0,162	0,084	0,08	0,518	0,187	0,092	0,08	0,314	0,167	0,081	0,128	405
C	0,28	0,121	0,078	0,07	0,358	0,14	0,091	0,076	0,232	0,101	0,086	0,089	405
D	0,234	0,101	0,074	0,069	0,317	0,114	0,085	0,085	0,171	0,08	0,08	0,069	405
E	0,19	0,085	0,072	0,069	0,228	0,095	0,082	0,075	0,121	0,085	0,091	0,076	405
F	0,142	0,098	0,074	0,084	0,165	0,102	0,137	0,095	0,093	0,097	0,094	0,095	405
G	0,112	0,094	0,067	0,073	0,1	0,087	0,098	0,076	0,102	0,073	0,074	0,075	405
H	0,09	0,117	0,106	0,099	0,107	0,085	0,162	0,072	0,094	0,075	0,092	0,072	405

Medium binding

	1	2	3	4	5	6	7	8	9	10	11	12	
A	0,532	0,229	0,081	0,061	0,877	0,421	0,141	0,071	1,399	0,352	0,132	0,062	405
B	0,395	0,128	0,073	0,06	0,644	0,188	0,09	0,062	1,469	0,281	0,121	0,062	405
C	0,273	0,093	0,068	0,064	0,456	0,11	0,083	0,059	0,964	0,153	0,102	0,058	405
D	0,216	0,077	0,063	0,064	0,323	0,091	0,073	0,06	0,69	0,148	0,09	0,061	405
E	0,134	0,074	0,064	0,061	0,204	0,076	0,068	0,061	0,382	0,09	0,078	0,059	405
F	0,095	0,064	0,063	0,058	0,14	0,078	0,072	0,062	0,214	0,081	0,083	0,059	405
G	0,076	0,065	0,058	0,057	0,1	0,068	0,069	0,067	0,134	0,074	0,075	0,059	405
H	0,08	0,065	0,065	0,06	0,096	0,068	0,065	0,059	0,122	0,068	0,073	0,066	405

Low binding

	1	2	3	4	5	6	7	8	9	10	11	12	
A	0,349	0,095	0,062	0,062	0,351	0,095	0,075	0,065	0,292	0,096	0,069	0,061	405
B	0,231	0,073	0,062	0,061	0,207	0,091	0,073	0,062	0,211	0,083	0,066	0,064	405
C	0,131	0,07	0,061	0,064	0,188	0,076	0,064	0,059	0,164	0,068	0,063	0,062	405
D	0,103	0,066	0,067	0,061	0,148	0,072	0,062	0,063	0,12	0,068	0,064	0,062	405
E	0,095	0,067	0,07	0,062	0,098	0,065	0,062	0,062	0,091	0,06	0,062	0,06	405
F	0,073	0,065	0,07	0,06	0,09	0,062	0,064	0,061	0,082	0,068	0,066	0,068	405
G	0,069	0,061	0,063	0,059	0,079	0,061	0,063	0,057	0,07	0,068	0,067	0,065	405
H	0,069	0,071	0,063	0,059	0,073	0,061	0,06	0,064	0,071	0,062	0,064	0,061	405

Figure 2.
Indirect ELISA to standardize the ligation of TcISP2r in 96 wells plates with different binding capabilities using anti-histidine antibody. TcISP2r histidine tailed protein, purified by histidine affinity chromatography, were ligated to plates of high, medium, and low binding capabilities as indicated in the figure. Columns 1 to 4 contain 1 ug of protein per well; 5 to 8, 2 ug; and 9 to 12, 5 ug. Columns 1, 5, and 9 started with 1 ug of anti-his antibody; columns 2, 6 e 10, started with 0,1 ug of anti-his antibody; colunms 3, 7, and 11, started with 0,05 ug of anti-his antibody; in columns 4, 8, and 12 no anti-his antibody were used. From a to H, anti-his antibodies were serially diluted in order of 2 (1:2; 1:4; 1:6; 1:8; 1:10; 1:12: 1:14; 1:16).

carbonate-bicarbonate buffer, pH 9.2. The plates were filled with 100 μL of buffer containing 1, 2, or 5 μg of protein and kept in the refrigerator for 16 hours. Subsequently, the plates were washed with 20 mM of phosphate buffer pH 7.4 and 0.05% of tween 20 and subsequently incubated with blocking solution (5% skim milk, 20 mM of phosphate buffer pH 7.4 and 0, 05% tween 20) for 30 minutes. Then, the blocking solution was removed and different dilutions of the anti-histidine monoclonal antibody (1 ug, 0.1 ug, and 0.05 ug/mL) produced in mice (Invitrogen) in 50 uL of blocking solution were added per well. Serial dilutions in the order of 2 of the anti-histidine antibodies were also made in columns A to H, followed by incubation for 2 hours at room temperature. After washing three times with 20 mM of phosphate buffer pH 7.4 and 0.05% tween 20, 0.1 ug/mL of the anti-mouse IgG second antibody, bound with alkaline phosphatase, was added to 50 uL of blocking solution and incubated for 1 hour at room temperature. The plate was then washed 3 times with 20 mM phosphate buffer pH 7.4 and 0.05% tween 20 and 2 times with 20 mM phosphate buffer pH 7.4 without tween 20. Reactions were developed with PNPP substrate for alkaline phosphatase (Invitrogen), according to the manufacturer's instructions and the plates were incubated for 30 minutes at room temperature and read in a spectrophotometer at a wavelength of 405 nm.

ELISA tests were performed in 96-well plates with medium binding capacity and three concentrations of TcISP2r protein (2, 5, and 10 μg). Recombinant protein binding was carried out for 16 hours in 100 uL of 0.1 M carbonate-bicarbonate buffer pH 9.2, in the refrigerator. Subsequently, the plates were washed with 20 mM of phosphate buffer pH 7.4 and 0.05% of tween 20 and subsequently incubated with blocking solution (5% skim milk, 20 mM of phosphate buffer pH 7.4 and 0, 05% tween 20) for 30 minutes. Then, the blocking solution was removed and 50 uL of serial dilutions of serum from 3 mice collected at 7-, 15-, and 60-days post-infection were added to the wells and the plate incubated for 2 hours at room temperature. After three washes with 20 mM of phosphate buffer pH 7.4 and 0.05% tween 20, 0.1 ug/mL of the anti-mouse IgG second antibody, bound with alkaline phosphatase, was added to 50 uL of blocking solution and incubated for 1 hour at room temperature. The plate was then washed 3 times with 20 mM phosphate buffer pH 7.4 and 0.05% tween 20 and 2 times with 20 mM phosphate buffer pH 7.4 without tween 20. Reactions were developed with PNPP substrate for alkaline phosphatase (Invitrogen), according to the manufacturer's instructions and the plates were incubated for 30 minutes at room temperature and read in a spectrophotometer at a wavelength of 405 nm.

3. Results and discussion

3.1 Phylogenetic inferences and TcISP2 origin and role in Chagas' disease

Maximum likelihood phylogenetic inference resulted in the tree represented in **Figure 3**, with *E. coli* ecotin as the outgroup and color-coded ISPs 1, 2, and 3. The tree topology strongly indicates that the ISP ecotin homologs have differentiated from each other a long time ago, and it is probable that at least ISP1 and ISP2 have been with these organism's genome at least since the split between the *Leishmania* and *Trypanosoma* genera.

Using the loci image generation software described in detail in the author's master thesis [43] resulted in the images in **Figures 4** and **5**, showing the full chromosomes and a zoomed-in area of interest respectively. **Figure 4** is only useful for comparing *Leishmania* records as to the overall position in the chromosome: ecotin homologs occur only in chromosome 15 of these species, and the data for other species is either incomplete or badly annotated, resulting in huge contig sequences. **Figure 5** clears the image a little, but data for *T. grayi* and *Leptomonas pyrrhocoris* sequences is still fragmentary.

The images show up to five ecotin homologs in various *Leishmania* species. This duplication was not reported in previous papers. Sequence data analysis and visual genomic context inspection give strong support to the idea that ecotin homologs suffered various duplications and/or multiple events of lateral gene transference before the differentiation of modern Trypanosomatida genera. Closely examining **Figure 5**, it can be seen that *Leishmania* spp. mostly retained all five ISP copies, while trypanosomes lost at least a few of them. In these figures, the conserved hypothetical coding sequences (*CHP1-3*) and *katanin-like* labels are accessory labels: they serve to identify the complete ecotin loci and were helpful to identify possible genomic evolutionary events involving ISP1, ISP2, and ISP3.

We know ISPs came from bacteria by horizontal gene transfer in Kinetoplastida because they appear in no other eukaryotes. The unanswered question is "how." Looking at **Figures 4** and **5** and keeping the cladogram in **Figure 3** in mind, we can form a hypothesis for how trypanosomatids acquired ecotin homologs. The next paragraph is speculative, but given the evidence, it probably is not too far off-base.

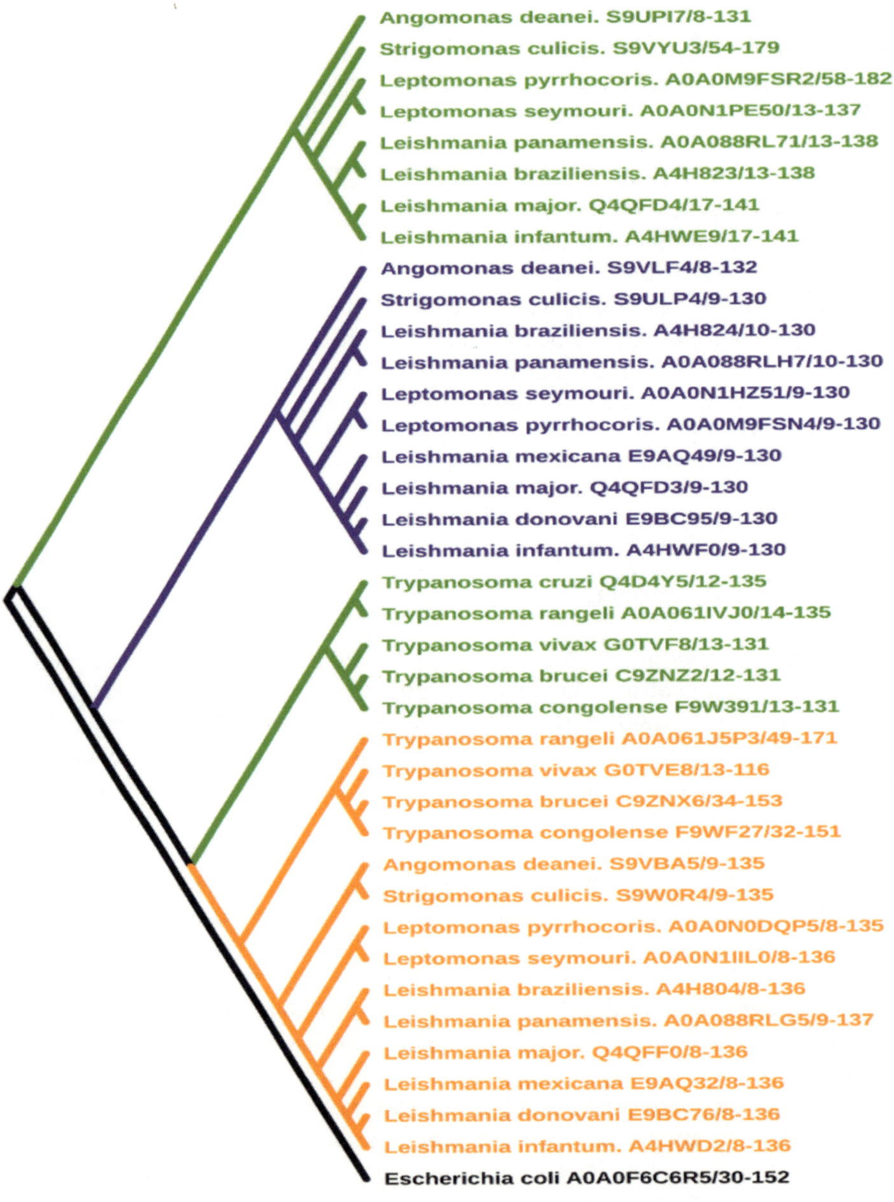

Figure 3.
Maximum likelihood cladogram of ecotin homologs (ISPs), with ISP1, labeled in orange, ISP2 labeled in green, and ISP3 labeled in blue.

The ancestor of all trypanosomatids either participated in multiple lateral gene transfers with ecotin-possessing bacteria or this event occurred only once and was followed by multiple gene duplications. If multiple gene transfers occurred, they probably happened no more than three times for ISPs 1, 2, and 3, and the additional ISP2 and ISP3 copies carried by *Leishmania* spp. are the result of a subsequent duplication. The positions of ISP1 and ISP2 in *T. brucei*, in the first and second ecotin loci respectively, with the ISP2 being probably homologous to *T. cruzi* ISP2, points to an early locus duplication, occurring before the two genera split. In this scenario, *Trypanosoma*

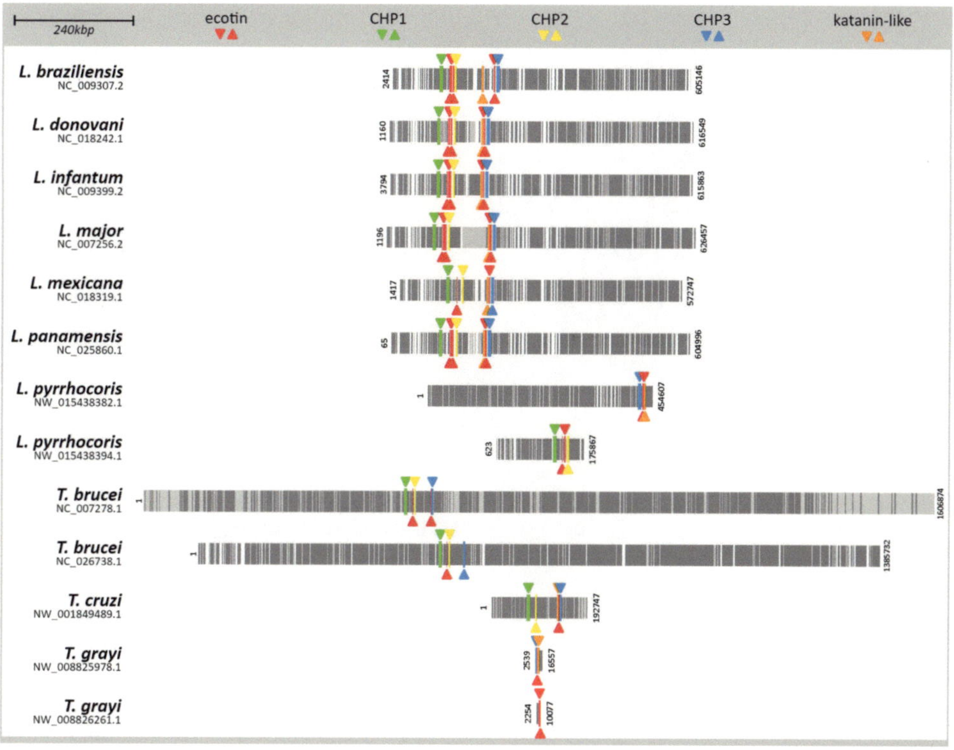

Figure 4.
Loci image generator result showing full GenBank records and all selected labels. Conserved hypothetical protein (CHP) 1 to 3, presenting highly similar amino acid sequences are represented by the same color. Seta direction indicates the orientation of the encoding gene according to genome annotation in GenBank.

spp. subsequently lost copies of the gene. Their sequences show a much more compact genome when compared to *Leishmania* spp. in the images presented, leading to the suspicion that more deletions occurred in *Trypanosoma* species than in *Leishmania*, which would lend credence to the idea that *T. cruzi* and *T. brucei* lost some of their ISP copies. A possible sequence of events based on this limited dataset is this: the common Trypanosomatida ancestor had three ISP copies in the first locus (at around position 120 kbp in chromosome 15), get either via lateral transfers with bacteria or via a single lateral transfer followed by contiguous duplication. The ISP2 and ISP3 ancestors in this locus then suffered a simultaneous duplication event, creating the second locus at around 190 kbp. Subsequently, various species lost some of these copies.

The preservation of ISP2 in almost all species is an interesting fact and makes sense given the ample evidence of its importance against hosts' immune systems. Another interesting fact is that *T. brucei* parasites preserved the ISP1 variant in all cases, while *T. cruzi* lost the ISP1 gene. Since ISP1 seems to be involved in the development of motility and flagellar development in promastigotes inside the insect vector in *Leishmania* species [31], this could be a reason for its preservation in *T. brucei* and loss in *T. cruzi*. These species are members of section Salivaria and Stercoraria, respectively, with different life cycles and methods of transmission. While *T. cruzi* is transmitted by hemipterans, with infecting parasites deposited with their feces on the vertebrate host, *T. brucei* lives in the salivary gland of dipteran insects and is injected by their proboscis like the *Leishmania* species. It could be that the ISP1 ecotin variant

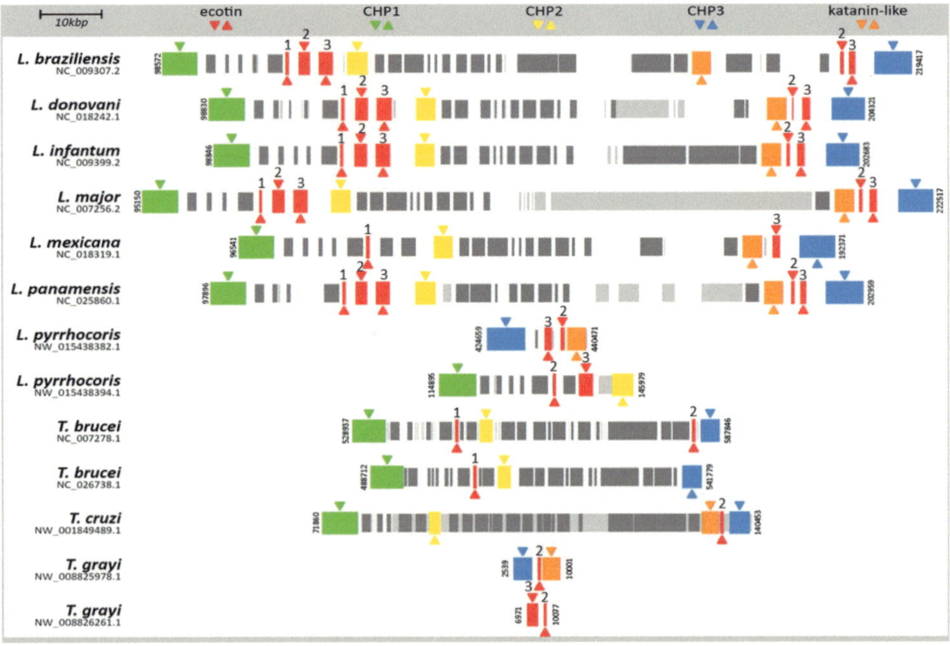

Figure 5.
Loci image generator result created with the same data as ***Figure 4*** *with a higher resolution and individual ISPs identified as ISP1, ISP2, and ISP3 with numbers; conserved hypothetical protein (CHP) 1 to 3, presenting highly similar amino acid sequences are represented by the same color; seta direction indicates the orientation of the encoding gene according to genome annotation in GenBank.*

gives some advantages to trypanosomatids with dipterans as their arthropod hosts. This association needs further investigation, resulting in data with potential public health applications.

These speculations are given to encourage further research. As tempting as it is to affirm their validity, our data set is very limited in scope and of very poor quality in some cases making bold affirmations. Automated genomic annotation can only go so far, and some of these sequences have errors, omissions, and other problems. Looking closely at the *L. mexicana* data in **Figure 5**, for example, it seems that the coding sequences between the first ISP occurrence and the CHP2 labeled gene should clearly be labeled as ISP2 and ISP3, but in the automated annotation, they appear as "*unknown proteins.*" Nevertheless, since the amount of available genomic data grows so fast, these speculations can be further developed as more data becomes available.

One thing this work clearly shows without a doubt is the ubiquity of large amounts of unreviewed genomic data online. The amount of retrievable information at very little monetary cost and using free-to-use bioinformatics tools is huge, and in this world of big data and exponentially falling sequencing costs, this fact will become more obvious as time passes. The next generation of budding biologists may well have to learn to program before they learn the names of all the plant and animal families.

T. cruzi presents only ISP2 in its chromosome 15, and its structural and biochemical characterization revealed high structural similarity with ecotin and strong inhibitory activity on human neutrophil elastase (NE) [44]. Ecotin appears to be a potent prokaryotic tool in evading the immune system. A classic example is that of the inhibition of NE: in humans, a serine peptidase produced in neutrophil granulocytes is one of the main immune defenses in combating pathogenic invaders. In bacteria, one of the ways of action of NE is the cleavage of outer membrane protein A (OmpA, from English outer membrane protein A) in phagocytosed gram-negative bacteria, hindering their multiplication [47, 48]. This makes ecotin an important target for pharmacological research [49].

3.2 TcISP2 is immunogenic in mice with chronic infection

To verify the immunogenicity of the recombinant form of the TcISP2 protein produced in *E. coli*, the indirect ELISA method was initially standardized. Recombinant proteins have different biochemical properties that determine the best conditions for coating ELISA plates with histidine-tagged TcISP2. Three different types of microplates were tested, each with a binding capacity and with different concentrations of recombinant protein. To assess the distribution of the protein in the wells, serial dilutions of mouse-produced anti-histidine antibodies obtained from Invitrogen were also analyzed. The results obtained showed that the medium binding capacity plate with 2 ug of recombinant protein per well presented the best results.

To confirm the infection of mice with the Y strain of *T. cruzi*, after 7 and 15 days, PCR was performed using the Tc121/122 oligos from a fraction of the clot obtained by puncturing the submandibular vein. The four mice infected after 7 days with the Y strain of *T. cruzi* were PCR negative, while the same mice were PCR positive after 15 days (**Figure 6**). After 60 days of infection, nucleic acids extracted from the cardiac lavage of two euthanized mice with infection confirmed by PCR and light microscopy were positive by PCR (**Figure 6**). These results indicate that blood parasites can only be detected 15 days post-infection in Black mice.

Serum from mice infected by *T. cruzi* strain Y, and collected after 7, 15, and 60 days, with results confirmed by PCR and light microscopy, was used in an ELISA experiment to evaluate the immunogenicity of TcISP2r. The results are shown in (**Figure 7**). The identification of TcISP2r was observed in the serum samples of mice

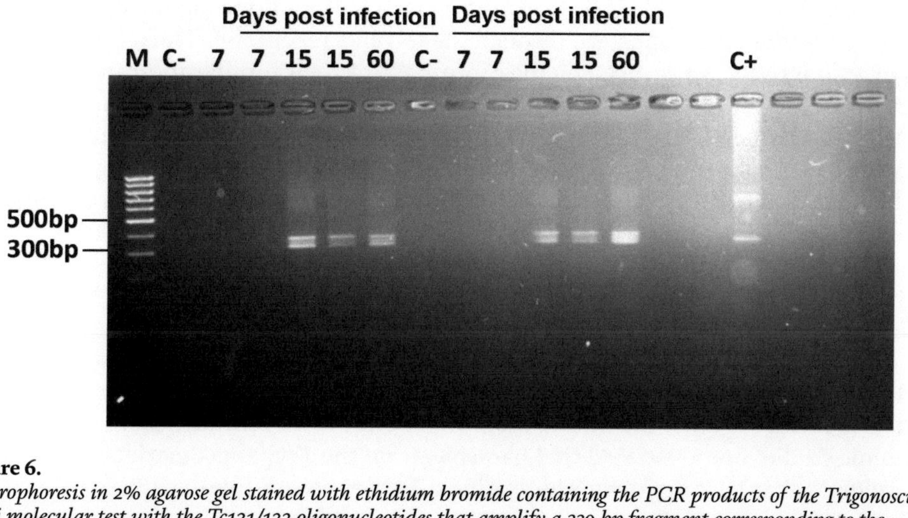

Figure 6.
Electrophoresis in 2% agarose gel stained with ethidium bromide containing the PCR products of the Trigonoscuta cruzi molecular test with the Tc121/122 oligonucleotides that amplify a 330 bp fragment corresponding to the gene encoding the parasite's kDNA. Blood clots of 4 infected mice after 7 and 15 days and the washing of cardiac tissue from 2 mice euthanized after 60 days of infection, were evaluated as indicated in the wells. C-, corresponds to the negative control of the PCR reaction; C+, corresponds to the positive control with genomic DNA obtained from T. cruzi of the Y strain; M – 100 bp ladder from synapse biotechnology.

A

Blank	Blank	Blank	Blank	Blank	Blank	Blank	Blank	Blank	Blank	Blank	Blank
2ug 1:10	2ug 1:10	2ug 1:10	2ug 1:10	5ug 1:10	5ug 1:10	5ug 1:10	5ug 1:10	10ug 1:10	10ug 1:10	10ug 1:10	10ug 1:10
2ug 1:20	2ug 1:20	2ug 1:20	2ug 1:20	5ug 1:20	5ug 1:20	5ug 1:20	5ug 1:20	10ug 1:20	10ug 1:20	10ug 1:20	10ug 1:20
2ug 1:40	2ug 1:40	2ug 1:40	2ug 1:40	5ug 1:40	5ug 1:40	5ug 1:40	5ug 1:40	10ug 1:40	10ug 1:40	10ug 1:40	10ug 1:40
2ug 1:80	2ug 1:80	2ug 1:80	2ug 1:80	5ug 1:80	5ug 1:80	5ug 1:80	5ug 1:80	10ug 1:80	10ug 1:80	10ug 1:80	10ug 1:80
2ug 1:160	2ug 1:160	2ug 1:160	2ug 1:160	5ug 1:160	5ug 1:160	5ug 1:160	5ug 1:160	10ug 1:160	10ug 1:160	10ug 1:160	10ug 1:160
2ug 1:320	2ug 1:320	2ug 1:320	2ug 1:320	5ug 1:320	5ug 1:320	5ug 1:320	5ug 1:320	10ug 1:320	10ug 1:320	10ug 1:320	10ug 1:320
2ug 1:640	2ug 1:640	2ug 1:640	2ug 1:640	5ug 1:640	5ug 1:640	5ug 1:640	5ug 1:640	10ug 1:640	10ug 1:640	10ug 1:640	10ug 1:640
Negative	D7	D15	D60	Negative	D7	D15	D60	Negative	D7	D15	D60

B

0,055	0,055	0,055	0,054	0,054	0,054	0,055	0,055	0,057	0,062	0,054	0,054
0,058	0,076	0,139	0,481	0,059	0,081	0,136	0,438	0,066	0,09	0,153	0,456
0,055	0,065	0,096	0,273	0,056	0,071	0,103	0,283	0,061	0,075	0,109	0,292
0,059	0,062	0,073	0,169	0,055	0,063	0,075	0,186	0,056	0,068	0,084	0,175
0,055	0,061	0,067	0,137	0,056	0,057	0,068	0,125	0,065	0,068	0,069	0,123
0,055	0,057	0,063	0,098	0,057	0,06	0,059	0,089	0,059	0,063	0,066	0,091
0,055	0,063	0,059	0,087	0,063	0,06	0,067	0,089	0,057	0,064	0,076	0,088
0,058	0,068	0,061	0,08	0,06	0,06	0,062	0,071	0,075	0,061	0,076	0,085

Figure 7.
Indirect ELISA test with different concentrations of TcISP2r and serum from mice infected with Trigonoscuta cruzi strain Y after 7, 15, and 60 days. A. Experimental design to verify the immunogenicity of TcISP2r in mouse sera collected 7, 15, and 60 days after infection with the Y strain of T. cruzi; negative control serum was obtained from uninfected mice; 2 μg; 5 μg and 10 μg are the amount of TcISP2r per well; B. absorbance results obtained after indirect ELISA test with alkaline phosphatase-labeled second antibody against mouse IgG, developed with P-nitrophenyl phosphate substrate.

60 days post-infection, suggesting an immune response against ISP2 from *T. cruzi* in the chronic phase of the disease. In ELISA tests, using mouse serum, the best protein concentration for antibody detection was also 2 ug.

The ELISA test revealed antibodies against TcISP2 in serum samples from *T. cruzi*-infected mice only after 60 days post-infection, during the chronic phase. The high activity of TcISP2 on neutrophil elastase indicates its inhibiting action on the immune system [44, 50]. In this way, inflammation would occur in infected organs and tissues during the chronic phase, when cardiomyopathy and mega syndromes (megaesophagus and megacolon) develop. Thus, we could infer that the activity of TcISP2 is to inhibit inflammatory activity and thus facilitate the colonization of tissues and organs by the parasite.

According to Faria et al. [33], ISPs are responsible for inhibiting the neutrophil elastase present in macrophages, through the toll-like receptor 4. Thus, cells with phagocytic activity can be used by the protozoan for their proliferation and escape from the immune system. In Chagas' disease, macrophages are infected and carry the parasite into tissues. The phagocytic action of macrophages is more relevant in tissues compared to other professional phagocytic cells, due to their ability to migrate from the bloodstream to different tissues and organs [51]. Thus, the TcISP2 can play an essential role in acute and chronic Chagas' disease.

4. Conclusions

Ecotin, a serine peptidase inhibitor (ISP), found first in *E. coli*, is a key factor in bacterial defense against the immunological barriers of vertebrate host organisms. Genomic studies demonstrated that parasites from the Trypanosomatida taxon are unique eukaryotic organisms harboring different ecotin-like encoding genes. Considering existence of trypanosomatida species with bacterial endosymbionts and the genomic context of ISPs demonstrated in this chapter, the evolutive origin of ecotin-like genes in trypanosomatids probably occurred by horizontal transfer from a symbiont bacterium, in a common ancestor of the clade, and this event was followed by successive duplications and losses that would explain the current pattern. *T. cruzi* present only one copy of ISP (TcISP) with high structural similarity to ecotin from *E. coli* and a strong inhibitory activity on human neutrophil elastase, indicating an exogenous activity and interaction with vertebrate host serine peptidases involved in the modulation of the immune system. The recombinant TcISP2 protein was immunogenic in a murine model, allowing the detection of antibodies in the chronic phase of *T.cruzi* infection, which suggested that this protein can also be tested as a target for serological diagnosis and for investigation of disease prognosis.

Acknowledgements

This work was funded by Fundação de Amparo à Pesquisa do Estado de São Paulo (FAPESP) (Grant number 2016/14514-4; and by UFABC. MMF and CMS were the recipient of a Master's scholarship from CAPES.

Conflict of interest

The authors declare no conflict of interest.

Additional information

Parts of this book chapter were initially presented in the Master thesis of Max Mario Fuhlendorf available on the UFABC library platform, titled Loci image generator and the evolution of trypanosomatid ecotin: customized software as a tool for evolutionary analysis, 2018, Programa de pós-graduação em Evolução e Diversidade. The thesis has not been peer-reviewed and published.

Author details

Carla Moreira Santana[1], Max Mario Fuhlendorf[1], Felipe Baena Garcia[1], Edmar Silva Santos[1], Ângela Maria Lourenço[2], Cristiane Castro Faccini[2], Abílio Augusto Fragata Filho[2], Aline Diniz Cabral[3] and Márcia Aparecida Sperança[1]*

1 Center for Natural and Human Sciences, Federal University of ABC, São Paulo, Brazil

2 Outpatient Clinic for Chagas Disease, Dante Pazzanese Cardiology Institute, São Paulo, Brazil

3 Department of Parasitology, Federal University of Uberlandia, Minas Gerais, Brazil

*Address all correspondence to: marcia.speranca@ufabc.edu.br

References

[1] Aguilar VHM. Reflections on Chagas disease in the Amazon. Memórias do Instituto Oswaldo Cruz. 2022;**117**:e200409chgsa. Epub 20220520. DOI: 10.1590/0074-02760210409chgsa

[2] Alvarez-Hernandez DA, Garcia-Rodriguez-Arana R, Ortiz-Hernandez A, Alvarez-Sanchez M, Wu M, Mejia R, et al. A systematic review of historical and current trends in Chagas disease. Therapeutic Advances in Infectious Disease. 2021;**8**:1-17. Epub 20210804. DOI: 10.1177/20499361211033715

[3] de Sousa PH, Scofield A, Junior PSB, Lira Dos Santos D, de Sousa Siqueira J, Chaves JF, et al. Chagas disease in urban and peri-urban environment in the Amazon: Sentinel hosts, vectors, and the environment. Acta Tropica. 2021;**217**:105858. Epub 20210212. DOI: 10.1016/j.actatropica.2021.105858

[4] Sarquis O, Carvalho-Costa FA, Toma HK, Georg I, Burgoa MR, Lima MM. Eco-epidemiology of Chagas disease in northeastern Brazil: Triatoma brasiliensis, T. pseudomaculata and Rhodnius nasutus in the sylvatic, peridomestic and domestic environments. Parasitology Research. 2012;**110**(4):1481-1485. Epub 20111007. DOI: 10.1007/s00436-011-2651-6

[5] Barbosa RL, Dias VL, Pereira KS, Schmidt FL, Franco RM, Guaraldo AM, et al. Survival in vitro and virulence of Trypanosoma cruzi in acai pulp in experimental acute Chagas disease. Journal of Food Protection. 2012;**75**(3):601-606. Epub 2012/03/14. DOI: 10.4315/0362-028X.JFP-11-233

[6] Brum-Soares LM, Xavier SS, Sousa AS, Borges-Pereira J, Ferreira JM, Costa IR, et al. Morbidity of Chagas disease among autochthonous patients from the Rio Negro microregion, state of Amazonas. Revista da Sociedade Brasileira de Medicina Tropical. 2010;**43**(2):170-177. Epub 2010/05/14. Morbidade da doenca de Chagas em pacientes autoctones da microrregiao do Rio Negro, Estado do Amazonas. DOI: 10.1590/s0037-86822010000200013

[7] Santos V, Meis J, Savino W, Andrade JAA, Vieira J, Coura JR, et al. Acute Chagas disease in the state of Para, Amazon region: Is it increasing? Memórias do Instituto Oswaldo Cruz. 2018;**113**(5):e170298. Epub 20180507. DOI: 10.1590/0074-02760170298

[8] Chung CH, Goldberg AL. Purification and characterization of protease so, a cytoplasmic serine protease in Escherichia coli. Journal of Bacteriology. 1983;**154**(1):231-238. Epub 1983/04/01. DOI: 10.1128/jb.154.1.231-238.1983

[9] Ivens AC, Peacock CS, Worthey EA, Murphy L, Aggarwal G, Berriman M, et al. The genome of the kinetoplastid parasite, Leishmania major. Science. 2005;**309**(5733):436-442. Epub 2005/07/16. DOI: 10.1126/science.1112680

[10] Kaufer A, Ellis J, Stark D, Barratt J. The evolution of trypanosomatid taxonomy. Parasites & Vectors. 2017;**10**(1):287. Epub 2017/06/10. DOI: 10.1186/s13071-017-2204-7

[11] Borghesan TC, Ferreira RC, Takata CS, Campaner M, Borda CC, Paiva F, et al. Molecular phylogenetic redefinition of Herpetomonas (Kinetoplastea, Trypanosomatidae), a genus of insect parasites associated with flies. Protist. 2013;**164**(1):129-152.

Epub 20120829. DOI: 10.1016/j.protis.2012.06.001

[12] Borges AR, Engstler M, Wolf M. 18S rRNA gene sequence-structure phylogeny of the Trypanosomatida (Kinetoplastea, Euglenozoa) with special reference to Trypanosoma. European Journal of Protistology. 2021;**81**:125824. Epub 2021/08/06. DOI: 10.1016/j.ejop.2021.125824

[13] Dollet M, Sturm NR, Campbell DA. The internal transcribed spacer of ribosomal RNA genes in plant trypanosomes (Phytomonas spp.) resolves 10 groups. Infection, Genetics and Evolution. 2012;**12**(2):299-308. Epub 2011/12/14. DOI: 10.1016/j.meegid.2011.11.010

[14] Sturm NR, Dollet M, Lukes J, Campbell DA. Rational sub-division of plant trypanosomes (Phytomonas spp.) based on minicircle conserved region analysis. Infection, Genetics and Evolution. 2007;**7**(5):570-576. Epub 2007/05/15. DOI: 10.1016/j.meegid.2007.04.002

[15] de Souza SSA, Catta-Preta CM, Alves JMP, Cavalcanti DP, Teixeira MMG, Camargo EP, et al. Expanded repertoire of kinetoplast associated proteins and unique mitochondrial DNA arrangement of symbiont-bearing trypanosomatids. PLoS One. 2017;**12**(11):e0187516. Epub 2017/11/14. DOI: 10.1371/journal.pone.0187516

[16] Motta MCM, Catta-Preta CMC. Electron microscopy techniques applied to symbiont-harboring Trypanosomatids: The Association of the Bacterium with host organelles. Methods in Molecular Biology. 2020;**2116**:425-447. Epub 2020/03/30. DOI: 10.1007/978-1-0716-0294-2_26

[17] Fraga J, Fernandez-Calienes A, Montalvo AM, Maes I, Deborggraeve S, Buscher P, et al. Phylogenetic analysis of the Trypanosoma genus based on the heat-shock protein 70 gene. Infection, Genetics and Evolution. 2016;**43**:165-172. Epub 2016/05/18. DOI: 10.1016/j.meegid.2016.05.016

[18] Rey L. Parasitologia. 4th ed. Rio de Janeiro: Guanabara Koogan; 2008

[19] Tyler KM, Engman DM. The life cycle of Trypanosoma cruzi revisited. International Journal for Parasitology. 2001;**31**(5-6):472-481. Epub 2001/05/04. DOI: 10.1016/s0020-7519(01)00153-9

[20] Hendriks E, van Deursen FJ, Wilson J, Sarkar M, Timms M, Matthews KR. Life-cycle differentiation in Trypanosoma brucei: Molecules and mutants. Biochemical Society Transactions. 2000;**28**(5):531-536. Epub 2000/10/25. DOI: 10.1042/bst0280531

[21] Votypka J, d'Avila-Levy CM, Grellier P, Maslov DA, Lukes J, Yurchenko V. New approaches to systematics of Trypanosomatidae: Criteria for taxonomic (Re)description. Trends in Parasitology. 2015;**31**(10):460-469. Epub 2015/10/05. DOI: 10.1016/j.pt.2015.06.015

[22] Alves JM, Klein CC, da Silva FM, Costa-Martins AG, Serrano MG, Buck GA, et al. Endosymbiosis in trypanosomatids: The genomic cooperation between bacterium and host in the synthesis of essential amino acids is heavily influenced by multiple horizontal gene transfers. BMC Evolutionary Biology. 2013;**13**:190. Epub 2013/09/11. DOI: 10.1186/1471-2148-13-190

[23] Jackson AP. Genome evolution in trypanosomatid parasites. Parasitology. 2015;**142**(Suppl. 1):S40-S56. Epub 2014/07/30. DOI: 10.1017/S0031182014000894

[24] McGrath ME, Gillmor SA, Fletterick RJ. Ecotin: Lessons on survival in a protease-filled world. Protein Science. 1995;**4**(2):141-148. DOI: 10.1002/pro.5560040201

[25] Yang SQ, Wang CI, Gillmor SA, Fletterick RJ, Craik CS. Ecotin: A serine protease inhibitor with two distinct and interacting binding sites. Journal of Molecular Biology. 1998;**279**(4):945-957. DOI: 10.1006/jmbi.1998.1748

[26] Eggers CT, Murray IA, Delmar VA, Day AG, Craik CS. The periplasmic serine protease inhibitor ecotin protects bacteria against neutrophil elastase. The Biochemical Journal. 2004;**379**(Pt 1):107-118. Epub 2004/01/07. DOI: 10.1042/BJ20031790

[27] Eggers CT, Wang SX, Fletterick RJ, Craik CS. The role of ecotin dimerization in protease inhibition. Journal of Molecular Biology. 2001;**308**(5):975-991. DOI: 10.1006/jmbi.2001.4754

[28] Jin L, Pandey P, Babine RE, Gorga JC, Seidl KJ, Gelfand E, et al. Crystal structures of the FXIa catalytic domain in complex with ecotin mutants reveal substrate-like interactions. The Journal of Biological Chemistry. 2005;**280**(6):4704-4712. Epub 2004/11/17. DOI: 10.1074/jbc.M411309200

[29] Seymour JL, Lindquist RN, Dennis MS, Moffat B, Yansura D, Reilly D, et al. Ecotin is a potent anticoagulant and reversible tight-binding inhibitor of factor Xa. Biochemistry. 1994;**33**(13):3949-3958. DOI: 10.1021/bi00179a022

[30] Eschenlauer SC, Faria MS, Morrison LS, Bland N, Ribeiro-Gomes FL, DosReis GA, et al. Influence of parasite encoded inhibitors of serine peptidases in early infection of macrophages with Leishmania major. Cellular Microbiology. 2009;**11**(1):106-120. Epub 20081029. DOI: 10.1111/j.1462-5822.2008.01243.x

[31] Morrison LS, Goundry A, Faria MS, Tetley L, Eschenlauer SC, Westrop GD, et al. Ecotin-like serine peptidase inhibitor ISP1 of Leishmania major plays a role in flagellar pocket dynamics and promastigote differentiation. Cellular Microbiology. 2012;**14**(8):1271-1286. Epub 20120508. DOI: 10.1111/j.1462-5822.2012.01798.x

[32] Ribeiro-Gomes FL, Moniz-de-Souza MC, Alexandre-Moreira MS, Dias WB, Lopes MF, Nunes MP, et al. Neutrophils activate macrophages for intracellular killing of Leishmania major through recruitment of TLR4 by neutrophil elastase. Journal of Immunology. 2007;**179**(6):3988-3994. Epub 2007/09/06. DOI: 10.4049/jimmunol.179.6.3988

[33] Faria MS, Reis FC, Azevedo-Pereira RL, Morrison LS, Mottram JC, Lima AP. Leishmania inhibitor of serine peptidase 2 prevents TLR4 activation by neutrophil elastase promoting parasite survival in murine macrophages. Journal of Immunology. 2011;**186**(1):411-422. Epub 20101122. DOI: 10.4049/jimmunol.1002175

[34] Ireland PM, Marshall L, Norville I, Sarkar-Tyson M. The serine protease inhibitor Ecotin is required for full virulence of Burkholderia pseudomallei. Microbial Pathogenesis. 2014;**67-68**:55-58. Epub 2014/01/28. DOI: 10.1016/j.micpath.2014.01.001

[35] El-Sayed NM, Myler PJ, Blandin G, Berriman M, Crabtree J, Aggarwal G, et al. Comparative genomics of trypanosomatid parasitic protozoa. Science. 2005;**309**(5733):404-409. Epub 2005/07/16. DOI: 10.1126/science.1112181

[36] Opperdoes FR, Michels PA. Horizontal gene transfer in trypanosomatids. Trends in Parasitology. 2007;**23**(10):470-476. Epub 2007/09/11. DOI: 10.1016/j.pt.2007.08.002

[37] Andrade IDS, Vianez-Junior JL, Goulart CL, Homble F, Ruysschaert JM, Almeida von Kruger WM, et al. Characterization of a porin channel in the endosymbiont of the trypanosomatid protozoan Crithidia deanei. Microbiology (Reading). 2011;**157**(Pt 10):2818-2830. Epub 2011/07/16. DOI: 10.1099/mic.0.049247-0

[38] Molyneux D. Neglected tropical diseases. Community Eye Health. 2013;**26**(82):21-24. Epub 2013/09/12

[39] Boratyn GM, Camacho C, Cooper PS, Coulouris G, Fong A, Ma N, et al. BLAST: A more efficient report with usability improvements. Nucleic Acids Research. 2013;**41**(Web Server issue):W29-W33. Epub 2013/04/24. DOI: 10.1093/nar/gkt282

[40] Gouy M, Guindon S, Gascuel O. SeaView version 4: A multiplatform graphical user interface for sequence alignment and phylogenetic tree building. Molecular Biology and Evolution. 2010;**27**(2):221-224. Epub 2009/10/27. DOI: 10.1093/molbev/msp259

[41] Darriba D, Taboada GL, Doallo R, Posada D. ProtTest 3: Fast selection of best-fit models of protein evolution. Bioinformatics. 2011;**27**(8):1164-1165. Epub 2011/02/22. DOI: 10.1093/bioinformatics/btr088

[42] Letunic I, Bork P. Interactive tree of life v2: Online annotation and display of phylogenetic trees made easy. Nucleic Acids Research. 2011;**39**(Web Server issue):W475-W478. Epub 2011/04/08. DOI: 10.1093/nar/gkr201

[43] Fuhlendorf MM. Loci Image Generator and Ecotin Phylogenetics: Customized Software as a Tool for Evolutionary Analysis. Santo André, Brazil: Federal University of ABC; 2018

[44] Garcia FB, Cabral AD, Fuhlendorf MM, da Cruz GF, Dos Santos JV, Ferreira GC, et al. Functional and structural characterization of an ecotin-like serine protease inhibitor from Trypanosoma cruzi. International Journal of Biological Macromolecules. 2020;**151**:459-466. Epub 20200218. DOI: 10.1016/j.ijbiomac.2020.02.186

[45] Sturm NR, Degrave W, Morel C, Simpson L. Sensitive detection and schizodeme classification of Trypanosoma cruzi cells by amplification of kinetoplast minicircle DNA sequences: Use in diagnosis of Chagas' disease. Molecular and Biochemical Parasitology. 1989;**33**(3):205-214. DOI: 10.1016/0166-6851(89)90082-0

[46] Telleria J, Lafay B, Virreira M, Barnabe C, Tibayrenc M, Svoboda M. Trypanosoma cruzi: Sequence analysis of the variable region of kinetoplast minicircles. Experimental Parasitology. 2006;**114**(4):279-288. Epub 20060530. DOI: 10.1016/j.exppara.2006.04.005

[47] Belaaouaj A, Kim KS, Shapiro SD. Degradation of outer membrane protein a in Escherichia coli killing by neutrophil elastase. Science. 2000;**289**(5482):1185-1188. Epub 2000/08/19. DOI: 10.1126/science.289.5482.1185

[48] Weinrauch Y, Drujan D, Shapiro SD, Weiss J, Zychlinsky A. Neutrophil elastase targets virulence factors of enterobacteria. Nature. 2002;**417**(6884):91-94. Epub 2002/05/23. DOI: 10.1038/417091a

[49] Myint SL, Zlatkov N, Aung KM, Toh E, Sjostrom A, Nadeem A, et al.

Ecotin and LamB in Escherichia coli influence the susceptibility to type VI secretion-mediated interbacterial competition and killing by vibrio cholerae. Biochimica et Biophysica Acta - General Subjects. 1865;**2021**(7):129912. Epub 2021/04/24. DOI: 10.1016/j.bbagen.2021.129912

[50] Levy DJ, Goundry A, Laires RSS, Costa TFR, Novo CM, Grab DJ, et al. Role of the inhibitor of serine peptidase 2 (ISP2) of Trypanosoma brucei rhodesiense in parasite virulence and modulation of the inflammatory responses of the host. PLoS Neglected Tropical Diseases. 2021;**15**(6):e0009526. Epub 20210621. DOI: 10.1371/journal.pntd.0009526

[51] van Furth R, Cohn ZA. The origin and kinetics of mononuclear phagocytes. The Journal of Experimental Medicine. 1968;**128**(3):415-435. DOI: 10.1084/jem.128.3.415